HOW MEN
CAN LIVE
AS LONG AS
WOMEN

HOW MEN CAN LIVE
AS LONG AS
WOMEN

SEVEN STEPS TO A
LONGER AND
BETTER
LIFE

THE SUMMIT GROUP

FORT WORTH, TEXAS

KEN GOLDBERG M.D.

This book is not intended to be a substitute for professional medical advice. The reader should regularly consult a physician regarding any matter concerning his health, especially in regard to any symptoms that might require diagnosis or medical attention. This book contains numerous references to actual cases the author has worked on over the years. However, names and other identifying characteristics have been changed to protect the privacy of those involved. Medical science is an everchanging field. Every effort was made to insure that the medical information contained in this book was the most accurate and current at the time of publication. Any mention in this book of actual products sold does not constitute an endorsement by the publisher or the author, except where noted.

THE SUMMIT GROUP
1227 West Magnolia
Suite 500
Fort Worth, Texas 76104

Printed in the United States of America

10   9   8   7   6   5   4   3   2   1

Library of Congress Cataloging in Publication Data
Goldberg, Ken.
    How men can live as long as women: seven steps to a longer and better life / Ken Goldberg.
        p. cm.
    ISBN 1-56530-025-4 : $22.95
    1. Men—Health and hygiene. I. Title
    RA777.8.G65 1993
    613'.04234—dc20   93-38419
                                                                    CIP

Cover design by Cheryl Corbitt.
Illustrations by Rusty Jones.

To Sharon—my wife, my friend, my love
forever and always.
And to my patients, thank you all so very much.

CONTENTS

If you smoke cigarettes, subsist on potato chips and beer, and exercise nothing more than your index finger on the remote control, it won't just ruin your health. When you become impotent because your arteries clog up, chances are your partner will feel as much pain and loss as you do. If you die young, you will not only create a widow. Perhaps even worse, you will have taught your children how to follow in your footsteps. It is a legacy that you don't want to leave.

You don't expect to be able to run the mile as fast when you're fifty as you could when you were twenty, and you shouldn't expect your penis to respond as quickly either. That doesn't mean you'll enjoy sex any less at fifty. Quite the opposite: You can enjoy it more when your body gives you time to relish the pleasure. You'll run that mile slower, but you might enjoy the scenery more.

Testicular cancer, for example, is most common in younger men, and most men don't see a doctor every year until they hit forty. Even then, that exam takes place on one day only. A lot of things can happen during the other 364 days of the year.

According to Dr. Louis Sullivan, former Secretary of Health and Human Services, about nine hundred thousand of the 2.2 million deaths in the United States each year are preventable. Your diet and exercise habits affect your likelihood of succumbing to fully four of the ten leading causes of death in men, and nine of the first ten are within your control to avoid.

American women make 130 million more doctor visits per year than men. Why? Not because they have more money or better insurance plans. Women are simply more attuned to taking care of themselves. But just going to the doctor isn't enough to give men back their full lives. Men hold attitudes about health—an entire catalog of male myths—that not only keep them from living longer, but also prevent them from fully enjoying the years they've got. Not until we throw off the notion that men are supposed to be bulletproof, to suffer through pain quietly and alone, will we really make progress at breaking down that seven-year barrier.

ACKNOWLEDGMENTS

T his book has been almost three years in the making, and more than 150,000 words have been put on paper at one time or another. Through numerous revisions, it has benefited from the talents of people too numerous to name, but at least the following special people have helped make what looked like an insurmountable task not only possible, but also fun. I am grateful:

To my wife for her patience, understanding, and support.

To my sons for their encouragement and understanding.

To my staff for assisting me with the many faxes, copies, and typing, and for their enthusiasm.

To Dave Schoonmaker, my friend and collaborator. This was certainly a labor of love. To his family for being so understanding of the time it took away from them.

To The Summit Group, especially Mark Hulme, Mike Towle, and Brent Lockhart. I couldn't ask for a better publishing company. Summit has allowed me so much input on every aspect of the project.

To Chris Tucker, my editor, for his energies and input in polishing and fine-tuning this project.

To Cheryl Long, for her diligence and expertise in fact checking the contents of this work.

To Gail Sheehy, Mike LaFavore, and Mike McGrath for their experience.

To my advisors and friends Barbara Buzzell, Helene Cohen, Sharon Fjordbak, Charles McBride, Laurey Peat, and Bob Reznik for their input and guidance.

Tonjia Roan, my practice administrator, deserves a special thanks for her support and effort, and for keeping the practice running.

To Dr. Neil Gordon, of the Cooper Institute for Aerobic Research, for his advice and expertise on Steps 4 and 5.

To Dr. Richard Honaker, family practitioner, friend and colleague, who offered tremendous help and guidance with many of the medical issues.

To Dr. Terry Bazzarre, senior nutrition science consultant of the American Heart Association for his advice and expertise regarding Steps 4 and 5.

To all those who wrote articles, books, and studies used for documentation in this book.

And definitely not last, my patients, who have provided the inspiration that made this book possible, especially those who were willing to share their experiences.

INTRODUCTION: HERE'S TO SEVEN MORE YEARS

(Read This First!)

Congratulations! The fact that you're reading these words means you want to take some control over your life and do what you can to get the most out of it. Even if reading this book wasn't your idea—maybe you got it as a gift, instead of a necktie—you've turned the first page on a new, longer, and better life.

This is a book about healthy, happy living for men, but much of it could apply equally well to women. We're not all that different, you know. What's the real difference between a man and a woman? Biologically, not much. A man has far more testosterone—the male hormone—in his blood than a woman does, and, of course, he develops different sexual organs and a different body shape.

In one regard, however, a man differs considerably from a woman: On average, his life is about seven years—almost 10 percent—shorter than hers!

Of course, it didn't take a team of scientists to figure that out. All you have to do is look at the crowds of seniors in Florida or Arizona—predominately female—to know that *something* about being male robs us of years that should be ours.

But what is that "something?" There's no biological law that says men must die earlier than women. Medical science has failed to find any reason why testosterone or a penis and testicles should cause us to fold early in the game. All the evidence says the problem isn't in the cards we're dealt; it's how we play them. It's how we live our lives that's causing us to die.

Here's a sad statistic: American women make 130 million more doctor visits per year than men. Why? Not because they have more money or better insurance plans. Women are simply more attuned to taking care of themselves.

I am a urologist who specializes in male health problems. The fact that men neglect their bodies is blatantly obvious to me every day. I was trained to correct those problems, but fixing the same ones over and over eventually became frustrating. I was like the mechanic who tries to salvage the car after the engine is burned up. The damage is already done.

Then, while running early one Saturday morning a few years ago, I was thinking about what I had to do that day. I had to tell three men in their fifties that they had advanced prostate cancer—that they were going to die. It was at that moment that I knew I had to do more than just treat male problems; I had to help *prevent* them. It was then that I knew I would write this book.

It would be easy for me to say that more visits to the doctor would save more men's lives. And that alone would help us catch some problems before they grow into death sentences. *But just going to the doctor isn't enough to give men back their full lives.* Men hold attitudes about health—an entire catalog of male myths—that not only keep them from living longer, but also prevent their full enjoyment of the years they've got.

Not until we throw off the notion that men are supposed to be bulletproof, to suffer through pain quietly and alone, will we really make progress at breaking down that seven-year barrier. Men can do it. I see the proof almost every day in patients who have changed their thinking about health:

MEN TALK: Jeff Stearns, age fifty-two

was fifty years old and thought I had life by the tail. I was competing in and winning triathlons, and was at the peak of my powers as a professional pilot. Then a routine airline physical turned up prostate cancer. Frankly, it sent me for a loop. I just couldn't believe this could happen to me.

"I spent quite a while in the dumps. It took the caring support of my wife, a fine doctor, and other men for me to figure out that I was actually lucky.

"First, the required annual physical found the cancer when it could still be successfully treated. On my own, I probably wouldn't have been having an annual physical.

"Second, I am a very fortunate man to have the woman I do. She convinced me that I was going to get through this, and her attitude built mine up. She encouraged me to keep running prior to the operation, and I think being in good shape had a lot to do with my recovery. She was there every step of the way. I got out of the hospital in five days, instead of the usual six or seven, and I was able to start exercising again within four weeks.

"Something else happened to me in the hospital, though. While I was recovering, other men with the same condition came to visit me. They told me what to expect, but more than that, they showed me that I wasn't alone and that I could get through this. We'd gone through something together, almost like war veterans, and it formed a bond. Now I return the favor. I'm an active member of Us Too, the prostate cancer support group.

"A year after the operation, I'm going strong. There's no recurrence of the cancer, and I'm back to competing in triathlons. Matter of fact, I took first place at the Male Health Center Fun Run a few weeks ago.

"But I assure you that I am not the same man I was before. I've always taken care of my body through exercise, and I thought that was enough. Sure, it helped me get through this, and I do believe in fitness, but I

also know for sure that we're in this together on this planet. We've got to help each other. It's added a whole new dimension to my life."

I want to stress again: There is no mysterious male curse, no testosterone tax, that dictates shorter lives for men. Nine of the leading causes of death in men—from heart disease to suicide—are preventable. Did you know that most cancers can be prevented? Or that almost all cancers can be cured if they're caught early enough? According to former Health and Human Services Secretary Dr. Louis Sullivan, more than nine hundred thousand deaths per year in the United States—about 40 percent of the total deaths—could be postponed by simple changes in life-style.

That's why I've organized this book, not in conventional chapters, but in seven *steps*—active steps you can take to improve and prolong your life. In the pages that follow, you'll learn:

- **how to read your family history for signs of future trouble**
- **how to find the best doctor and get the best care**
- **how to understand results of medical tests and physical exams**
- **how to eat right and exercise for best effect**
- **how to ward off cancer, heart disease, and the other eight leading causes of death for men**
- **how to be sure you enjoy sex throughout your life**
- **how to avoid ruining your life with a sexually transmitted disease.**

These are steps to a longer life. But just as important, they are steps to a *better* life. By following the steps in this book, you'll do far more than live longer. You'll enjoy those extra years to the maximum. After all, living an extra seven years doesn't mean much unless you're healthy enough to travel, fish, play golf, and do the other things you have looked forward to during your working years.

And one of those things, of course, is sex. Far too many men think that loss of potency is an inevitable part of aging, that we have to give up the great joys of good sex as we move past forty, fifty, sixty . . . .

Well, let me assure you that your penis does not wear out. If you take care of your body by eating well, exercising, and having regular sex with a loving partner, it should continue to serve you throughout your years.

Impotence, you see, is just another form of disability that strikes people who don't take care of themselves. Dr. Sullivan, again, tells us that two-thirds of long-term disability could be prevented. One researcher, Dr. Lester Breslow from the University of California at Los Angeles, has found in a twenty-year study that people who practice good health habits live longer and have markedly less disability than those who don't. Take another of my patients as an example:

MEN TALK: Harry Sullivan, age sixty

I was a health disaster. At fifty-five years of age, my cholesterol was over three hundred; I was thirty pounds overweight, and, to be brutally honest, I was impotent. My wife and I hadn't had sex in years. Without ever even talking about it, we'd just given up.

"Of course, it wasn't like I just forgot about that part of my life and went on with the rest. I didn't really feel like a complete man, and my career was suffering, too. If you can't perform in the bedroom, you can't perform in the board room, either.

"By the time I finally got some competent medical attention, my circulatory system was too far gone for any of the easy fixes—but I was able to get help. What I had to do, beyond getting medical care, was make myself over with a new diet, an exercise program, a solid relationship with my doctor, and a whole new view of how to live.

"I've got a new zest for life now. I watch what I eat and I walk four miles every day, rain or shine. My cholesterol is under two hundred and I've lost the extra pounds. Believe me, I feel ten years younger than I did five years ago.

"Best of all, I think my relationship with my wife is the best it's been in our thirty-five years of marriage. It's not just the sex, though, that's really good again. But aside from the sex, we enjoy each other's company more than ever. Need I say that my career has taken a successful turn, too?"

Harry demonstrates the most important kind of changes we'll deal with in this book—changing the way we think about ourselves. As men, we face an uphill battle against the messages we receive from our culture about what manhood should be. We're raised to compete and perform, instead of to cooperate and enjoy mutual successes. We learn that real men don't talk about how they feel, let alone actually express an emotion. We don't cry. We're supposed to be tough—to be able to take pain "like a man." Is it any wonder we consider going to the doctor an admission of weakness? And what about the most fundamental aspect of our masculinity—our sexuality? For that, our culture provides us with a set of fantasy role models—the Hollywood superstuds, the professional athletes. Comparing ourselves with them, we always come up short.

The overall message our culture offers men is that manhood is a precarious condition—it's constantly threatened by outside influences and must be defended by building barriers. In fact, however, the steps to a longer and better life require us to break down those barriers and step beyond those narrow roles:

A man can be a partner, and that involves much more than an erection and healthy sperm. It's sharing obligations, concerns, and emotions; being there to listen and to support; being honest and responsible; and taking pleasure in his partner's pleasure.

A man can be a father, and that involves much more than providing food and shelter. He can be a role model and set new standards for our culture. He can be compassionate and concerned; and he can educate.

And finally, a man can be a fellow man, and that involves much more than teasing and taunting each other, and sharing sexual boasts in a locker room. It means extending a hand to those who need help; talking honestly to one another and sharing feelings; and learning to cooperate rather than compete.

I f you can blend the knowledge available in this book with a new attitude about yourself as a man, you'll get what every man really wants most— more control over his own life. Your body will no longer be an adversary that threatens to let you down. It will become a tool you work with to enjoy life more.

You'll also find that taking care of yourself is a way of life rather than a set of hurdles to leap. The seven steps in this book are not absolutes. It's not a matter of doing them perfectly to get the results. You'll do better sometimes than others, which is perfectly normal. I like a beer and a hot dog at a ball game, and I enjoy sharing a glass of wine at dinner with my wife. This book does not outlaw fun. Many of us overindulge sometimes, and we shouldn't punish ourselves for it. All that matters is that we get back on track.

There's an old saying: "If I'm not for me, who will be for me?" No one should care more about your health than you do. So take the seven steps. You'll be glad you did.

1

**Taking Charge
of Your
Personal Health**

HOME IMPROVEMENT

MEN TALK: John Wellington, age thirty-four

I t all happened so quickly, I hardly had time to think about it. I got a call from my younger brother in mid-July saying that he had testicle cancer, and that the doctor had said he should let me know, because it runs in families.

"At the time, I wasn't totally ignorant about testicle cancer. The doctor who did my last physical mentioned that I ought to check myself. But he didn't tell me how or how often, so I really wasn't sure what I was doing. I suspected something might be wrong because one of my testicles was larger than the other. But I had no pain, so I put off making an appointment to be checked.

"When my brother called, though, I didn't hesitate. I called my doctor immediately. He referred me to a urologist who examined me and reported bad news. He said that based on how the testicle felt—there was a fair-sized hard lump—and the fact that my brother had testicle cancer, I probably had it too. More tests confirmed the diagnosis, and I was scheduled for surgery four days later.

"The surgery to remove the cancerous testicle was pretty easy, really. I went in at seven in the morning and was home by noon. I took five days off from work— there was some swelling, which I put ice packs on— and I never even used up the pain medication the doctor gave me. After a day, I didn't need it.

"It's only been ten days since the surgery, but I'm feeling fine. Tests showed that the surgeon got all the cancer, so I shouldn't have further trouble. Just to be sure, though, I'm scheduled for radiation treatments next week. My brother says he didn't feel much of anything when they gave him radiation, and the treatments only lasted about ten minutes.

"This hasn't been fun, but I know how lucky I've been. My cancer turned out to be somewhat more advanced than his, and if it had gone much longer untreated, I could have been in real trouble. Because I wasn't doing an adequate job of checking myself, it was only the warning from a relative that saved me from complicated surgery or even death. I certainly intend to pass this information along to my sons and grandsons."

What's the most important message in this book? Simple. Good health isn't something you *receive from* a doctor; it's something you *develop with* a doctor. It's your body, and nobody cares more about it than you do. *You* have to take an active role in your health if you want to live a longer, more satisfying life.

Think of it this way: Would you drive your car until the tread on the tires wears through completely and they go flat? Of course not. It's much cheaper (not to mention safer) to check tread wear every so often and avoid nasty blowouts. Your body is much the same way, only the stakes are even higher. Ignore it, and something unexpected and unpleasant is likely to happen.

Like every automobile model, every human body has its strengths and weaknesses. Knowing what diseases your predecessors have had is as valuable as knowing the recall history of your type of car. Listen to your body and get help when it's got a problem—just as you would head straight for your mechanic if your car started making unusual noises.

Your power to prevent most diseases—and to notice those you do get before they become serious—far exceeds any doctor's ability to cure you once you're really sick. I can help you know *what* to look for based on your family history, and I can help you learn *how* to look for it. But the first line of defense in quality medical care is in your hands.

What's Up Your Family Tree?

Altogether, there might be as many as fifty-seven hundred diseases with a familial link, and each of us carries genes that predispose us to developing, on average, eight of them.

Baseball player Ken Griffey, Jr., race-car driver Al Unser, Jr., and country singer Hank Williams, Jr. are not the only ones who are carrying on a family tradition. Your height, your hair color, and—to some extent—even your life span, are part of your genetic inheritance, handed down in the strings of DNA your mother and father, and their mothers and fathers, passed on to you.

As medical science draws closer to unraveling the mysteries of genetics, we find more and more ways in which our chromosomal heritage affects the lives we lead. You are made from a wondrous, but limited, menu of available characteristics. Some of the offerings on that menu, unfortunately, can be hazardous to your health.

Altogether, there might be as many as fifty-seven hundred diseases with a familial link, and each of us carries genes that predispose us to developing, on average, eight of them (according to Mary Jo Harrod, Ph.D., of the University of Texas Southwest Medical Center in Dallas). I have little doubt that as more of the body's nearly one hundred thousand genes are mapped, more inheritable diseases will turn up.

Before you start cursing your great-grandfather, keep in mind that being genetically susceptible to a certain disease does not mean that you absolutely will get that disease. Our genes dictate our destiny only in a few relatively rare cases such as cystic fibrosis, hemophilia, and Huntington's chorea. In one of the most famous examples, folk singer Woody Guthrie was born

Many forms of diabetes run in families, but having a diabetic dad is no death sentence. Recent research has shown that life-style changes such as a low-fat diet and regular exercise can help head off diabetes and also control it without insulin.

with Huntington's, which took his life in 1967. For years, his son, Arlo, has lived in uncertainty about whether he had inherited the disease.

In the vast majority of cases, however, a genetic tendency in a family only means that you are more likely to develop the disease. Many forms of diabetes run in families, but having a diabetic dad is no death sentence. Recent research has shown that life-style changes such as a low-fat diet and regular exercise can help head off diabetes and also control it without insulin. And, of course, it's no secret that diet and exercise can protect you from inheritable circulatory disorders such as heart disease and high blood pressure. It's less well known that one form of high cholesterol is an inherited problem that's particularly dangerous to men. Half of men with familial hypercholesterolemia die by age sixty.

It's clear, then, that knowing your family history—putting together a genetic scouting report—gives you power. What our forebears have left us isn't so much a risk of disease as it is fair warning to take care of ourselves. By reading your genealogy carefully, you can see trouble coming and head it off at the pass. Use the form on the following page as a guideline when conducting your family research.

Your Family History

Definitions: *Immediate family* includes father, mother, grandparents, brothers, and sisters. *Second-degree relatives* are uncles, aunts, and cousins.

1   What have your immediate family members died from, and at what age?

_____

_____

_____

2   What have your second-degree relatives died from, and at what age?

_____

_____

_____

3   What medical problems do or did they have?

_____

_____

_____

4   What medications do or did they take?

_____

_____

_____

5   What habits, good and bad, do or did they have?

_____

_____

_____

6   What kind of surgeries or other hospitalizations have they had?

_____

_____

_____

7   What kind of exposures to toxins have they had at work or elsewhere?

_____

_____

_____

Prostate Cancer

Diseases With Family Ties

For men, there's no better example of a predictable disease than prostate cancer. In the last year, studies at Johns Hopkins University have shown that a man with a family history of prostate cancer runs an increased risk of getting it himself. The study indicated that men in families of more than one affected relative—especially a case before age fifty-five—the risk is about 50 percent, or about four times the risk for men that have no affected relatives. Also, prostate cancer can be inherited from either side of the family.

Learning that your father, or an uncle or grandfather from either side of the family had prostate cancer might strike you as the worst sort of news—just short of a death sentence. Not so. Knowing you're likely to get prostate cancer is far better than not knowing you have it. And you need all the warning you can get, since prostate cancer most often has no detectable symptoms until it's too late. But it's one of the slowest-growing cancers, and if diagnosed early, it's nearly always curable. Sometimes, however, it's so slow growing that we don't even treat it at all.

Recently, a fifty-eight-year-old man came to see me during a prostate cancer screening. His brother, who was three years older, had just been diagnosed with prostate cancer. My patient seemed fine and had no symptoms or problems. But when we did a rectal examination, we found a small lump in his prostate. A biopsy showed prostate cancer. As we talked, he told me that his father had died of prostate cancer and that his grandfather probably also had it.

This man was at extremely high risk for this cancer, yet he had never made the knowledge about his family history work for him, or for his sons or nephews. In any family where there is a history of prostate cancer, it's very important that all the males get screened starting at age forty with rectals and the PSA (prostate specific antigen) blood test. For men without a family history of prostate cancer, according to a Washington University study, an annual digital rectal exam beginning at forty and regular blood tests after fifty will catch most prostate cancers.

Testicular Cancer

The other main male cancer—testicular—also has a strong basis in family history. First, men who had undescended testicles when they were young are at a significantly greater risk. Ask your parents if you belong to that group. At least as significant, recent research in Great Britain has shown that men whose fathers have had cancer of the testicles are at four times the risk of developing it themselves.

And the genetic tie appears even stronger between brothers: When one has the disease, the risk to the other is nearly ten times the normal rate. At least as disturbing, genetically based testicular cancer:

- **appears to start at an earlier age in each new generation,**
- **is more likely to affect both testicles, and**
- **is more likely to spread to other organs.**

If anything, early detection—which is much more likely if you know you're at risk and check yourself regularly—is more important with testicular cancer than with prostate cancer. Testicular cancer grows faster than prostate cancer, so the self-exam I'm going to describe (on page 12) is especially important. But as with prostate cancer, a testicular cancer found early can be cured completely and relatively easily. Your family tree is your early-warning system.

Colorectal Cancer

Some types of colorectal cancer are known to be passed on genetically, and just last year researchers identified a specific genetic abnormality that can predispose a person to develop colorectal cancer. In a few years, it's possible that you'll be able to undergo testing to determine your risk, but for now your relatives are still your best clue. As we'll discuss in-depth later, a healthful life-style can help disarm this killer.

A low-fat, high-fiber diet has been shown in numerous studies to reduce risk, while eating grilled (especially barbecued) meats, which contain compounds called nitrosamines, increases the risk.

Here again, early detection is vitally important. You should regularly have a sigmoidoscopy (visual examination of the rectum and lower large intestine with a flexible instrument) and, if you have a family history or other risk, you should have a regular colonoscopy to catch polyps (precancerous growths) before they become cancers. (Intervals and descriptions for these tests are spelled out in the next step.)

Talking to Your Family Tree

I'm all in favor of the growing popular enthusiasm for genealogy we've seen over the last decade or two. Modern-day living does have a tendency to separate us from our heritage. But we need to know more about our roots than just birthdays, migrations, and notable achievements.

Talk to your parents, grandparents, and other relatives about what ailed your ancestors. Granted, it's not easy to probe into such delicate matters with a maiden aunt or an aging grandfather. Your success will depend on your being tactful but firm, and letting them know just why this is so important to you and your offspring.

Talk to your parents, grandparents, and other relatives about what ailed your ancestors. Granted, it's not easy to probe into such delicate matters with a maiden aunt or an aging grandfather. Your success will depend on your being tactful but firm, and letting them know just why this is so important to you and your offspring.

Press them to be specific. (A prostate problem, for example, might be different from prostate cancer.) And, if you have access to them, check death certificates for causes. Over the years, medicine has become much more precise and terminology has changed, but your doctor can help you sort out what's important.

Keep a record of what you discover about your ancestors' health, so that medical history becomes as much a part of your family tree as military history. Genetic heritage is a vital part of the legacy your forebears left you. Be sure you make the most of it. And be sure you pass this scouting report on to your sons and daughters.

Self-Tests for Self-Protection

Quick Inspections

Self-tests are the core of basic routine body maintenance. They're quick inspections (at least monthly) that you should no more ignore than you would ignore periodically checking your engine's oil or the air in your tires. They take only a few minutes per month, but they can add years to your life—healthy years that are well worth living.

Women heard the message about self-tests long ago. They're accustomed to inspecting their breasts regularly, and that habit carries over to greater overall attention to their bodies. Most men, however, seem to view self-inspection (and self-preservation!) as an admission of vulnerability. Despite that common male attitude, I can assure you that we are not bulletproof—not even when we're young. Testicular cancer, for example, is the most common solid cancer in younger men, and most men don't see a doctor every year until they hit forty. Even then, that exam takes place on one day only. A lot of things can happen during the other 364 days of the year.

Just getting help when we hurt isn't enough. By the time symptoms announce themselves loudly, it might be too late. You need to be looking for problems *before* they become noticeable. By keeping tabs on your own body between doctor visits, you significantly increase the chances of detecting a serious condition while it's still easy to treat. You'll recover more quickly, you might avoid chemotherapy or radiation, and your health-care costs will be much lower. And the fact is, for some diseases, all the surgical expertise in the world will do you no good if things have gone too far. Self-tests can save your life.

Self-examination *is* good medicine, but it's also a good attitude. Getting to know the fleshy enclosure in which you live will further increase the sense of control you have over your life.

Testicular Self-Exam

Though few young men know about it, testicular cancer happens to be the number-one solid cancer in males under the age of thirty-five. We've made great advances in curing testicular cancer—over 90 percent can be successfully cured—but early detection makes the job much easier, avoiding chemotherapy and major surgery.

Of all the self-exams men should be performing, the testicular self-exam is unquestionably the most vital for guys under forty. Simply put, you don't see the doctor often enough for him to have a decent chance of catching testicular cancer before it's too late. It's your responsibility to find it and save your own life.

> *Every man who's reached puberty should examine his own testicles at least once per month. The best time is when you're in the shower, since your scrotum relaxes from the warmth.*
> (See Figure 1)

Every man who's reached puberty should examine his own testicles at least once per month. The best time is when you're in the shower, since your scrotum relaxes from the warmth. Refer to the following three things when checking your testicles (*See Figure 1 on page 12*).

By examining yourself regularly, you get a sense of what's normal. If you feel a lump, see your doctor *immediately.* This is not something to report at your next physical. I've examined guys with testicles the size of grapefruits who claimed they just noticed the problem the night before. I don't know how noticeable such a thing might be, but I can tell you that even the fast-growing testicle tumors don't swell to the size of softballs overnight.

Sores on Your Penis

After you've checked your testicles in the shower, take a minute to examine the skin on your penis. Note any sores or lumps and mention them to your doctor. A sore could be something as simple and unthreatening as an irritated hair follicle—or as se-

Testicular Self-Exam (*Figure 1*):

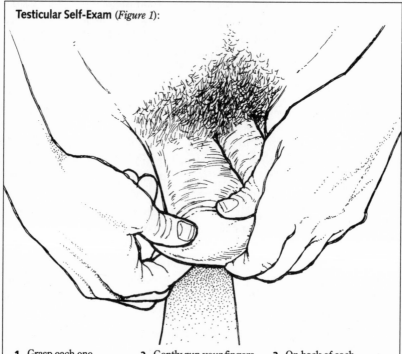

1 Grasp each one between your thumb and first two fingers, with your thumb behind.

2 Gently run your fingers around the circumference of each testicle while looking for lumps or hard places. The testicle should feel much like a hard-boiled egg without its shell—only smaller.

3 On back of each testicle, where your thumb is, you might find a lump called the epididymis, but the rest of the surface should be smooth and rubbery.

rious as a sexually transmitted disease, or the beginnings of penile cancer. You be the (private) investigator, and let your doctor be the judge.

Unusual Skin Changes

In an average lifetime, a man has about a 20-percent chance of getting skin cancer. There are three main types. Basal cell and squamous cell can usually be cured without too much difficulty, but the third—malignant melanoma—can be deadly.

Over the last forty years, all types of skin cancer have become much more common, perhaps in part because sunlight has become more intense owing to damage to Earth's protective ozone layer. Many skin cancers get their start when your skin is damaged by the sun, and increased ultraviolet radiation—which the ozone layer normally screens out—raises that risk.

It's important for you to limit your exposure to sunlight whenever you're outside for extended periods by:

* **using sunscreen (with an SPF—sun protection factor—of at least 15),**

* **wearing a hat, and**

* **wearing long sleeves.**

But it's equally important to watch for precancerous changes in your skin. Check your skin at least once a month, and see your doctor if you have a sore that doesn't heal, or a mole-like growth. If you notice such a growth, apply the following A-B-C-D test:

A   **asymmetrical (not round) shape, or**

B   **borders that are irregular, or**

C   **color variation across its surfaces, or**

D   **diameter bigger than a pencil eraser.**

If the growth exhibits any or all of these characteristics, you could have a problem.

At the Male Health Center in Dallas, we have offered a cancer screening program in which we do all the examinations appropriate for a man's age, according to the American Cancer Society. One forty-eight-year-old man came to see us anticipating a prostate check. As we did the cancer screening, we found a black spot on his foot which was biopsied and determined to be malignant melanoma. He went to a dermatologist who removed a small amount of tissue and found that the cancer had been eradicated. The man is now totally normal, doing fine—and doing his self-exams.

Just remember A, B, C, and D as you check your entire body—from the soles of your feet, to your back, to your scalp. If at all possible, ask your partner to examine hard-to-see areas, and return the favor. Needless to say, you should be even more diligent if you have a parent or grandparent who has skin cancer or if you have spent a lot of time outside.

Breast Cancer—Not Just Her Concern

In the popular imagination, breast cancer is exclusively a woman's disease. Not so. Although breast cancer occurs much less often in men than it does in women, there are almost a thousand cases of male breast cancer reported each year, and it can be just as deadly when it strikes a man. While writing this book, I diagnosed cases in two men. They were lucky, because early detection is very important with breast cancer. Unfortunately, because men are much less aware of the problem than women, few examine themselves, so the prognosis usually is not good by the time it's detected.

At least once a month, examine your chest by gently rubbing the area around your nipples with the tips of your fingers to reveal lumps. (Men are more likely to get cancer around the nipples, because they have less flesh elsewhere.) Note the following factors:

- The tissue should all be of the same consistency.
- There should be no changes from one month to the next.
- There should be no pain when you press gently.
- Squeezing the nipple should not produce a discharge.

Down in the Mouth: Guarding Against Oral Cancer

Many people have the mistaken impression that chewing tobacco products is somehow safer than smoking cigarettes. But a quick glance at oral-cancer statistics would quickly cure them of that notion—and, believe me, oral cancer is a miserable way to die. Baseball players, many of whom use oral tobacco products, have unusually high rates of mouth, throat, esophagus, and stomach cancers.

Although cancers of the mouth and throat are very rare among people who don't use tobacco products, you should know that persistent sores in the mouth are not to be ignored.

The minor leagues have already banned chewing tobacco, and the majors are likely to follow suit in the next few years.

Although cancers of the mouth and throat are very rare among people who don't use tobacco products, you should know that persistent sores in the mouth are not to be ignored. To check yourself, simply run your tongue around your gums searching for any persistent sore spots. Those that don't disappear or begin to heal up within a few days should be examined by your doctor or dentist. (And by the way, your dentist should be examining your mouth for potential cancers every time you have a checkup.)

Swollen Glands

Lymph glands, located in your neck, armpit and groin, are particularly sensitive indicators of trouble because, as part of your immune system, they act as a filtering system within the body. Foreign substances, whether they be cancers or various infections, are trapped in the lymph nodes. So check them regularly for signs of swelling and tenderness. You'll have trouble finding them when everything is fine, but a swollen node will stand up and demand attention. If you find one, see your doctor to find out what's causing the inflammation.

Putting Your Finger on the Pulse

Heart rate isn't a diagnostic procedure for any particular disease, but an abnormally low or high pulse can represent a problem. It wouldn't hurt to check your pulse every month or so when you first wake up in the morning. Report any significant changes to your doctor. Also be on the lookout for irregularities in your pulse. Variations could be normal, but might signal one of a group of conditions called arrhythmias. Later on, as explained in Step Four, pulse rate will also become an important part of your exercise program. Knowing your resting heart rate will be helpful, and being able to take your pulse quickly will be important for proper training. Here's how:

1   Place your index and second fingers on your neck between the side and the front. You'll feel an indentation where you'll pick up a strong pulsing.

2   Count the beats for fifteen seconds, and then multiply that number by four to calculate your pulse rate per minute.

Monitoring Your Blood Pressure

High blood pressure (called hypertension) is the single greatest risk factor for cardiovascular diseases such as heart attack and stroke, and it's frighteningly common. Nearly a third of all men over eighteen have it. That's why I'm devoting a good deal of space to the problem, especially in Step Three.

Simply put, high blood pressure means that your entire circulatory system has to work harder to deliver blood where it's needed. If your blood pressure remains consistently elevated, it can damage blood vessels and increase the strain on your heart—causing it to enlarge.

You've probably heard your doctor or nurse refer to your blood pressure (BP) as two numbers, one "over" the other. The first, higher number is called the systolic pressure—the pressure when your heart pumps. Diastolic pressure, the lower number, is the resting pressure between heartbeats.

Normal blood pressure depends on age and even on gender, but we usually consider anything in the vicinity of 130 over 80 or less is okay. People do vary considerably, though—both individual to individual, and from one time to another—so there's no strict level that's normal or abnormal. Check the chart in Step Three.

Many doctors diagnose mild hypertension when diastolic pressure rises to between ninety and one hundred, or a systolic rises to between 140 and 160. Likewise, they may declare a person hypertensive if diastolic pressure goes over one hundred or systolic pressure climbs past 160. We don't know all the things that can cause high blood pressure, but we know that genetics, salt, stress, and excessive alcohol cause it in some people. The problem is readily treatable, as long as you know you have it. Your doctor—or his nurse—will check your blood pressure almost every time you visit his office. If it turns out to be above normal, that *might* mean you have a problem.

Why "might?" That's because one blood pressure reading doesn't tell your doctor what your blood pressure is *on average*. It might be that your blood pressure jumps up only when you go to the doctor's office—what we call "white coat syndrome"—and that it's just fine the rest of the time. In my experience, most men who see me for potency problems have elevated blood pressure resulting from the understandable stress that comes from bedroom problems and the fear of discussing it with a doctor. Their blood pressure frequently returns to normal after

	How to Take Your Own Blood Pressure
1	Wait for at least thirty minutes after exposure to stimulants that raise blood pressure, such as caffeine, eating, exercise, and cold.
2	Urinate or have a bowel movement, if necessary.
3	Sit in a chair next to a table positioned so you can rest your arm comfortably on the table top with the palm up. Relax for five minutes.
4	Wrap the cuff around your upper arm so that its lower edge is about an inch above your elbow, and the two tubes are positioned to the inside and directed toward your hand. Tighten it enough so that it won't slide off.
5	Place the gauge on the table so you can see it easily.
6	Slip the cup of the stethoscope up under the cuff on the inside, and put the earpieces in your ears.
7	Tighten the valve on the squeeze bulb, and pump the cuff up until the gauge reads about 180.
8	Loosen the valve slightly, so that the pressure begins to bleed off by two or three millimeters per second.
9	When the pressure drops to between 150 and 120, you'll begin to hear a tapping noise. The pressure where you first hear it is your systolic pressure.
10	As the pressure continues to bleed off, the tap will gradually become a swishing noise and then a less distinct tap. The reading at which you can last hear any noise measures your diastolic pressure.

we've dealt with their problems and they've gotten used to talking with me.

If your doctor does find that your blood pressure is above normal, you should have it checked a few times in a non-threatening situation. Drop by the fire station or see your nurse at work if you have one. Or, if you like, buy a blood-pressure cuff (called a sphygmomanometer) and check your own pressure regularly. By measuring your blood pressure at different times of the day, you can learn how much of the time it's elevated, and you might even get an idea what's causing it to go up (if it's up only at the office, for example).

> *If your doctor does find that your blood pressure is above normal, you should have it checked a few times in a non-threatening situation.*

Glucose Tests for Diabetes

If you have a family history of diabetes or your doctor finds that you have diabetic tendencies, he or she might recommend that you use an over-the-counter, blood-glucose diabetes test regularly. This simple device—which you can buy at a local pharmacy—gives you a quick reading of how well your system is handling sugar. Values over 150 should be of concern.

Understand, though, that diabetes is serious business. It's not something you should try to diagnose or treat yourself. Diabetes can lead to serious kidney problems, and diabetics often become impotent because of nerve damage. If you have any of the common symptoms of diabetes—thirst, persistent weariness, or frequent urination—you should see your doctor and find out for sure if you are diabetic.

> *Diabetes can lead to serious kidney problems, and diabetics often become impotent because of nerve damage.*

These days, diabetes can usually be controlled or even reversed without injections of insulin. In fact, a conscientious diet and regular exercise are often enough to return diabetics to a normal life.

Stamping Out Impotence

You might wonder why any man would need to do a self-test for impotence. Surely, there's not too much of a question about whether you have the problem or not. True, but the source of a potency problem has much to do with overall health—as I explain later in the section on potency. Erection problems are always a symptom of some other difficulty, and a simple self-test can help you find out what's causing it.

During the night, while they sleep, almost all potent men have two to four erections lasting fifteen to thirty minutes each. We're not even aware of them unless we happen to wake up with an erect penis.

To find out if you're having nighttime erections, just wrap a strip of postage stamps (no need to spring for first class here, any denomination will do) snugly around your penis and glue one end to the other. If you have an erection during the night, the swelling will break the stamps along a perforation.

I've recommended the stamp test for many men who came to me for help with their impotence. They were astonished to find that they were indeed having nocturnal erections. And by the way, although many men awaken with "pee hard-ons" during the night, there's no physiological connection between erections and the need to urinate. It's just coincidence. The need to urinate awakens you, and you then notice you're erect. I've never met a man who told me he got a full erection when he had to urinate during the day.

Mixing Work and Pleasure

Finally, remember that there's no reason why self-exams should be unpleasant or even tedious—especially if you make them a regular ritual with your partner. Caring for each other physically is one important aspect of any relationship. And with a little imagination, you can turn self-exams into partner-exams—and a whole lot of fun.

Flashing Red Lights

Listen To Your Body

Paying attention to what your body is trying to tell you is the motorist's equivalent of noticing flashing red lights on the dashboard. Heed them, and you can head off problems before they become seri-

Paying attention to what your body is trying to tell you is the motorist's equivalent of noticing flashing red lights on the dashboard.

ous. When you see the oil-pressure light come on, you get help right away. You don't wait until your next scheduled maintenance to do something about it. Likewise, you can't afford to ignore problems with your body until you can get around to seeing a doctor.

Although self-tests are mandatory if you're going to discover quiet problems before they become noisy, many other ailments announce their presence loud and clear. Please, please, don't ignore their messages.

The Seven Warning Signs of Cancer

According to the American Cancer Society, there are seven basic warning signs every person should be on the watch for:

1 **a change in bowel or bladder habits, such as**
   a thinner stool
   a change in color of urine or stool, or
   a change in frequency

2 **a sore that doesn't heal**

3 **unusual bleeding or discharge:**
   in your ejaculate
   in your stool
   in your urine, or
   coughing up blood

4 **a lump or thickening anywhere on your body, looking especially:**
   under your arm, or
   in your breasts

5 **indigestion or difficulty swallowing**

6 **obvious change in a wart or mole**

7 **nagging cough or hoarseness**

Chest Pain

Pain, especially during exertion—ranging from a sense of tightness in the center of the chest to very severe pain that might radiate to the neck or down the left arm—is a sign that arteries are unable to supply enough blood to the heart. A number of other less dangerous conditions—heartburn, for example—might mimic angina. Most angina-like conditions don't ease when you rest. If your pains continue, further testing is in order.

Angina, or *angina pectoris* in medical circles, is a symptom of heart disease, but many people are able to reduce their angina by losing weight, stopping smoking, getting regular exercise (directed by a doctor), and changing their diet. Drugs also might reduce symptoms, but when less invasive methods fail, surgery might be necessary.

Because "heart attack" has such an ominous ring, it's at the top of that long list of things we believe will happen only to other people—never to us. A friend of mine, a man who regularly played racquetball, ran and lifted weights, was home by himself one day when he began experiencing some heaviness in his chest. It wouldn't go away. He tried one friend, then called me in desperation.

I told him I was concerned and insisted he get to the emergency room. He was reluctant to call 911, so he drove himself to the hospital, where doctors found that he was having a heart attack. Had he ignored the symptoms, who knows what might have happened? The mortality rate is highest during the first few hours of a heart attack.

Dizziness, Fainting, Heavy Sweating, Shortness of Breath

Although pressure or pain in the chest lasting more than a few minutes is one of the most common symptoms of a heart attack, some people have severe heart attacks without ever experiencing severe chest pain. Besides that sensation that there's a truck driving over your chest, you might become very dizzy, sweat heavily, and become nauseous—or even faint. A very common sign of heart attack in older people is severe shortness of breath. The symptoms we have mentioned might, of course, signal other problems, such as asthma or lung disease, but they're a cause for a doctor visit in any event.

Impotence

We'll talk in detail about this in Step Six, although you should consider a persistent problem involved with getting or maintaining erections to be a symptom of other health problems. In more than half of all cases, impotence stems from a physical problem, such as clogged arteries, high blood pressure, or diabetes. More than a quarter of the men who see me for erection difficulties have high cholesterol, and researchers at the University of California at Los Angeles have found that about a quarter of all men who see a doctor for a potency problem caused by reduced blood flow have a heart attack or stroke within five years. Even when emotional problems are at the bottom of things, a limp penis is still a sign of another problem that should and can be treated on its own.

In more than half of all cases, impotence stems from a physical problem, such as clogged arteries, high blood pressure, or diabetes.

Stroke

Stroke is the leading cause of disability in the United States, but awareness of stroke symptoms is sadly lacking. Early treatment of stroke is at least as important as it is for heart attack, so remember these warning signs:

1   sudden weakness or numbness of one side of the face, an arm, or a leg

2   sudden dimness or loss of vision, particularly in one eye

3   loss of speech or the ability to understand speech

4   sudden severe headache without other cause

5   dizziness, unsteadiness, or falls, especially along with any of the previous symptoms

Diabetes

The most common form of diabetes develops gradually during the adult years. Symptoms become progressively worse, until diabetes is full-blown and potentially life-threatening. With a few simple lifestyle changes, diabetes can be controlled or even reversed, but it's much easier if you catch it in its early stages. You should talk to your doctor about diabetes if you have two or more of the following symptoms:

1 regular or constant thirst

2 frequent need to urinate

3 fatigue

4 unexplained weight loss

Headaches

Every man gets some throbs and twinges between the ears now and then. Some of these pains—following a big party, for example—are pretty easy to explain. Others are more mysterious and persistent. These are the ones that have us hearing the faint message ("Brain tumor . . . brain tumor") with each thunderclap in our temples.

Rest assured that the great majority of headaches mean nothing more than stress, sinus infection, or fatigue. But they can also be the warning drumbeats of high blood pressure. If a headache plagues you for an unusually long time—more than a few days—you should check with a doctor.

Bleeding and bruising easily can be a sign that you're deficient in the platelets that are important in blood clotting.

Bruising and Bleeding

If you cut yourself shaving and it won't stop bleeding, or if you seem to bruise every time you bump something, your body might be sending you an important signal. Bleeding and bruising easily can be a sign that you're deficient in the platelets that are important in blood clotting. These symptoms can also be related to anemia, cancer, liver problems, or vitamin deficiency.

Abdominal Pain

A pain that begins in the middle of the abdomen and migrates across to the lower right part of your abdomen could be a sign of appendicitis. Other causes of abdominal pain include hernias, if the pain is down low, and ulcers if the pain is higher.

The Sweats

Should you awaken some night drenched with sweat—and there's nothing wrong with your air conditioner—you could have an infection. In the worst-case scenario, heavy night sweating can indicate tuberculosis or AIDS.

Coughing

Coughing is one of those physical reactions that is linked to a staggering number of problems—some trivial and some quite serious. Coughing and constant hoarseness could mean that you, like President Bill Clinton, have a problem with gastroesophageal reflux disease, in which acid from the stomach comes back up the esophagus, often during sleep, and irritates the throat. Persistent coughing could also be a warning sign of pneumonia or lung cancer. If you've got these symptoms and you haven't had a nagging cold lately, give your doctor a call.

Fatigue

Everybody knows that "Thank God It's Friday" fatigue that comes from an unusually hard week of work. But most of us bounce back fairly fast after a night of rest. If you sense that you're abnormally tired for no discernible reason, you might be experiencing anemia, or heart and lung problems. As we noted above, the heart attack can be a sneaky beast; sometimes, persistent fatigue is the only symptom that alerts us to the problem.

Weight Loss

Dropping pounds—is that something to worry about? Yes, if you're not trying to lose weight or not doing some extraordinary physical work that eats up the calories. If you lose more than five pounds without a good reason, look into it. Rapid weight loss can indicate cancer and a number of other major illnesses.

Feeling Down for Extended Durations

We all have occasional periods of the blues, but depression is a different matter. If you lose interest or pleasure in most normal activities and have one or more of the following symptoms, you should be seeking help for a medical problem that can be cured:

1 poor appetite

2 disturbed sleep

3 lack of energy

4 loss of interest in sex and other pleasurable activities

5 feelings of worthlessness and futility

6 suicidal thoughts

Write Down Your Symptoms

Whenever your body sends you a message, write down what happened. Memories are not nearly as accurate as the written record. In a small notebook, jot down what seemed to bring on the problem—anything might be helpful, even if it doesn't seem important at the time—and what else was going on while you had the symptom. Take your notes with you when you see the doctor. Here are some things to ask yourself while jotting down your notes:

Symptoms Checklist	
1	How and when did the symptoms start?
2	Have the symptoms changed in frequency, severity, or duration?
3	What makes the symptoms better or worse (activity, eating, time of day)?
4	How long do the symptoms last?
5	On a 1-to-10 scale, how severe are the symptoms?
6	Are there any new or additional symptoms?
7	What are you doing when the symptoms occur?
8	Does any medication (including nonprescription) lessen the symptoms?
9	Have you ever had these symptoms before?
10	What do you think is causing the symptoms?
11	Are any family members or friends experiencing these same symptoms?

It's Your Car—Drive It Properly!

Taking a hand in your own health doesn't stop with the end of this step or with the end of this book. Being knowledgeable about your body is your right and responsibility. But to continue to do the best job, you must consider reading this book to be just the beginning. I've made every effort to give you the most current information in this book, but medicine changes at an amazing pace. Keep up-to-date with the latest medical developments through your local paper, news magazines, television, and maybe even a subscription to a publication dedicated to developments in preventive health care. This is a beginning—one that will give you the groundwork to continue learning and improving your life.

Taking care of your body gives you assurance and control, just as knowing that your car is well-maintained gives you confidence on the highway. Like mechanics, doctors help with expertise, but there is no one you should trust more than yourself to monitor your health.

> *Like mechanics, doctors help with expertise, but there is no one you should trust more than yourself to monitor your health.*

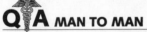 **MAN TO MAN**

QUESTION	ANSWER
When should I do self-exams, and how long should I expect them to take?	To answer your second question first, examining your testicles, penis, breasts, mouth, and skin should take no more than a couple of minutes—a small amount of time to dedicate monthly to better health.

When to perform self-exams, however, is a more difficult question. Women have a monthly cycle to remind them when to examine themselves. But we men aren't so lunar. I suggest you pick out a day that's already marked by something else that month, and always do your exams on that day. Maybe it's the day you pay your mortgage or make a car payment. Maybe it's a day with a significant number for you—seven for good luck? The important thing is to have a reminder and do those tests.

QUESTION	ANSWER
When I examine my testicles, there's a small lump in my scrotum, but not on a testicle. It's been there as long as I've been examining myself, and it hasn't changed in size or consistency. Should I be concerned?	There are a number of conditions that can produce small lumps in your scrotum, most of which aren't serious. If the lump is definitely not on or in a testicle, causes no pain, and remains the same size, you don't need to make a special appointment to see your doctor. Just mention it to him next time you're in touch. But if you're not sure, better safe than sorry. See your doctor.

QUESTION	ANSWER
I've heard the expression first- and second-order relatives and understand that it makes a difference in risk of disease, but I don't know what these terms mean. For instance, what order relative is an uncle, and how much should I worry if he's had prostate cancer?	A first-order relative is a parent, brother or sister, or child. Because your genes are more than 50 percent common, your risk is highest if a first-order relative has had a disease. Second-order relatives are grandparents or aunts or uncles. Your risk is lower if only a second-order relative has had a disease. Then again, the actual ratio of risk varies, depending on what genes you actually have in common and how genetic risk is carried on your chromosomes.

QUESTION	ANSWER
How do bad genes make a person get cancer or some other disease?	First off, you don't actually inherit the cancer itself. So it's not really a matter of having "bad" genes. Rather, we think—and there's still a lot to learn here—that people inherit certain genetic characteristics that make it easier for cancer to take hold.

For example, everyone has what we call tumor suppresser genes—specific bits of DNA that resist growth of tumor cells. Some people might be deficient in a particular suppresser gene that normally controls a particular kind of cancer cell. So, if there is |

some insult to their system—radiation, toxic chemicals, etc.—they're more likely to develop a cancer.

There are also substances in the body called growth factors, which, if over-produced because of a genetic defect, might cause tumor cells to grow too rapidly for the body to eliminate them.

The real point here is that a genetic predisposition to cancer or another inheritable disease does not mean you will get it. By taking care of yourself, you can overcome the increased odds your genes have given you, and live a long and healthy life.

QUESTION	ANSWER
My grandfather had prostate cancer when he passed away—he'd had it for a number of years—but the official cause of death was pneumonia. If I'd just looked at his death certificate, I never would have known. Is that often a problem?	True, the official cause of death might not mention the disease that sent the person into decline. That's why it's so important to talk to relatives who would know. In your grandfather's case, though, prostate cancer actually may not have had much to do with his death. Prostate cancer is a slow-growing malignancy—especially in men in their later years—and many men live with it for years without being troubled. In fact, autopsy studies show that more than 50 percent of men over the age of eighty have prostate cancer, but that's not what usually kills them.

QUESTION	ANSWER
What can I do to reduce the risk of my child inheriting a disease?	Since we're a little short of being able to genetically engineer people (thank goodness!), there's nothing you can specifically do to alter your genes. No drugs or other treatments will make a difference. But there's much you can do to reduce the risk to your children. First, you shouldn't consider trying to conceive a child until you've quit smoking, stopped drinking, gotten in decent shape, and generally put your own physical health in good order. Smoking, in particular, can affect the quality of your sperm, and tobacco byproducts can be transported into the woman's egg by sperm.

Then, once you have a child, teach him or her good health habits: diet, exercise, self-exams, regular checkups, etc. And, perhaps most importantly, set a good example for healthy living yourself.

HOTLINES	
Center for Science in the Public Interest	· **(202) 332-9110**
Health Risk Appraisal (Center Disease Control)	· **(404) 329-3452**
Library of Medicine	· **(301) 496-6095**
National Center for Health Statistics	· **(301) 436-8500**
National Headache Foundation	· **(800) 843-2256**
National Institute of Health	· **(301) 496-4000**
Office of Consumer Affairs	· **(202) 690-7694**
Peoples Medical Society	· **(800) 624-8773**
Skin Cancer Foundation	· **(212) 725-5176**

2

Finding the Health Partner Who Is Right for You

DRAFTING DR. RIGHT

MEN TALK: Ellis Hughes, age sixty-eight

Y*ou wouldn't believe how many doctors I went through before I found one who was really interested in helping me with my problem.*

"Okay, I'll be perfectly honest here. I've had an erection problem for more than ten years. I could get it up, but it wouldn't stay up long enough for intercourse. I saw a urologist in 1983—a doctor with an excellent reputation in my town. I told him what was going on, and he actually told me, 'Ellis, that's just what happens to us when we put on a few years. You can't expect it to work like it did when you were twenty.'

"Fortunately, I'm pretty stubborn, and my wife is even more stubborn. We didn't accept his explanation. I was sure that there was somebody out there who could help me. I tried three more urologists and didn't get much more help from them than I got from the first one. One gave me testosterone shots, but that didn't help. Another one said maybe it was psychological, and I should see a psychiatrist.

"Finally, one day I was in my car listening to the radio and heard a doctor being interviewed about prostate cancer. Right away, I could hear that he had a different attitude from the physicians I'd seen before. He talked about lots of different treatment options, and said that there were options for any problem. And he said that no matter how alone you might feel with your problem, there are lots of other men out

there who are going through the same thing.

"As soon as I got home, I called his office and made an appointment. He was very straightforward with me. We'd start with the least invasive option and move up to the next step if that didn't work. He said that it might take a few tries, but he was sure that we could do something about my erections.

"To make a long story short, we went through the whole list of simple treatments, and in the end I decided to have a penile implant. If you haven't heard of it before, a penile prosthesis probably sounds kind of gruesome. But it wasn't that big a deal surgically, and think about the alternative. I haven't a single regret, except that I was unable to find the right doctor sooner, and ended up spending a decade without a vital part of my life. I didn't give up, but if I had it to do over again I would have been even more persistent about getting the right care."

'm confident I don't have to convince you to see a doctor. Sure, American women do make 130 million more doctor visits each year than men. That's one reason they live an average of seven years longer. But if you have read this far, you are convinced.

Rather than waste space preaching, I want to tell you how to find the doctor who is right for you. And most important of all, I want to talk with you about a new approach to health—a new philosophy that will help you live longer and happier, get far more for your health-care dollar, and give you control over your own health.

I call it the health partnership. It goes without saying that your health professional must be a well-trained, skilled, and conscientious healer. But healing is not enough. To really get your money's worth, you need a *partner* who wants to help you learn how to *stay* healthy. It's much less expensive and less painful to avoid getting sick than it is to be healed. Again, remember the idea of preventive maintenance. We've got to stop thinking of visiting a doctor as a

> *To really get your money's worth, you need a partner who wants to help you learn how to stay healthy. It's much less expensive and less painful to avoid getting sick than it is to be healed.*

last-ditch effort to keep from keeling over. Ideally, you and your health partner will often talk about *staying* well, not just getting well. You'll talk about winning more years of life, years you can spend free from high blood pressure, high cholesterol, and other leading health problems many men face.

This new approach is not really that radical. Look at it this way. In the first step, we talked about doing self-tests on your body—the physical equivalent of regularly checking the air in your car's tires. Let's pull the car out into the driveway again and see if it's got another lesson for us to learn. What about the brakes? Do you have to plow through the back wall of your garage before you get someone to check the brakes? Of course not. Most of us don't even wait until we hear those horrible, expensive grinding noises, because we know it's much cheaper to replace the pads before the rotors get ruined.

I don't know about you, but I'm pretty picky about who works on my vehicles. I like an upfront explanation of what's going to be done. And if there's a problem, I expect to be told why the part broke and what I could have done to prevent it from happening. Why should your working relationship with your health partner be any different?

Finding Dr. Right

Over the next ten years, we're going to see a lot of changes in health care. Economics and common sense demand it. With politicians and pressure groups all talking about health-care reform, nobody can predict exactly how the system will change, but one thing is pretty clear: To be sure you get quality care at a reasonable price, you're going to have to be a smart medical consumer.

You see, the old saying got it right: Knowledge is power. When you learn what to expect from a physician, you'll have power regardless of how the system might change. If you end up selecting your own doctor, you'll know what to ask (and expect) to be sure you're getting the best. On the other hand, if a health maintenance organization (HMO) or some similar organization picks the doctor, you've still got to be well informed. Armed with the right knowledge, you'll know what care you should be getting. And if you don't get it, you can demand it.

However the health-care system changes, it's going to be a buyer's market. Back when there were much fewer doctors than we have today, people were pretty much obliged to accept what they got, especially if they lived in smaller towns where choices were more limited. That often meant long delays in getting appointments, multi-hour sits in the waiting room (why do you think they called it that?), and mediocre care.

That time is over. (Well, except for those irritating waits at certain doctors' offices. More on that later.) The laws of supply and demand—more doctors vying for the available patients—are creating competition. And, since insurance companies are looking to individuals to pay more of the bill—and that will only increase in the future—we're all becoming more conscious of how our money gets spent. You are the customer, and you should expect the best.

For many of you, this is going to require a change in attitude. People who grew up thinking of doctors as remote, omnipotent authority figures might have a hard time saying something like, "Hey, Doc, shouldn't you check my prostate?" But if your doctor neglects to do something that's necessary in your situation, you've been cheated. It's that simple. You wouldn't let your mechanic or your plumber get away with shoddy work—and it's much easier to get a new car or kitchen sink than to get a new body! As you build your health-care team, don't draft any players whose minds aren't in the game.

By the time you get to the end of this step, I want a new, more assertive you. Remember the old 1960s' slogan, "Question authority"? You don't have to carry

> *Knowledge is power—the power to stay healthy longer—so let's talk about what you should know and how to find it out.*

a protest sign, but be willing to question. Be ready, if the situation demands it, to say, "Whoa, stop. Please give me my bill and I'll be on my way." Knowledge is power—the power to stay healthy longer—so let's talk about what you should know and how to find it out.

Don't think of this as talking back to your doctor. Really, it's talking *with* your doctor. When you have a real health-care partner who treats you more as an equal, you'll be less likely to hear what some of my patients suffering from erection problems have heard from doctors: "Well, what do you expect? You're getting older." That's usually followed with the admonition to "Go home and relax." (The problem, of course, is that the wrong part of the body is relaxing!)

Some of this advice might sound overly ambitious, as if I'm counseling perfection. Well, being ambitious for the right things is not a sin. And there's nothing wrong with aiming for perfection, although we all fall a little short. You probably set lofty goals and high standards for your work at the office. But no man is bulletproof, no matter how much we think we are, and you don't want to wait until it's too late to recognize you have a problem. When the quality of your life is on the line, it's a good idea to be just as demanding.

Setting up a Get-Acquainted Visit

Sometimes, just a phone call to a doctor's office can give you a pretty good idea about this prospective partner. Ask the receptionist to mail you a brochure, assuming they have one. That will give you a free look at the scope of services and the policies of the practice, as well as a hint at the attitudes of the doctor and staff. During the same conversation, ask about fees—and don't settle for vague estimates. Expect a price range and if you end up being charged more, request an explanation. How much does a full examination cost, and how much are follow-up visits? How long does a typical visit last?

If possible, though, it's better to meet your would-be health partner face-to-face. At the very least, any doctor should welcome you to his or her office for a look-around. And many M.D.s will be happy to give you a short introduction—from a brief handshake to a few minutes of conversation, depending on schedules—without charging you. (For billing purposes, doctors can't charge you for a quick introductory visit, because that would affect your insurance reimbursement for a subsequent *complete* examination.

You won't get much time on this reconnaissance mission, but if you know what you're looking for and add your impressions of the facility and the staff, you'll be pretty clear about whether you've met "Dr. Right."

What should you look for? To start with, be aware that diplomas—universities attended and certifications earned—don't mean as much as they once did. All medical schools are fully accredited and the vast majority offer a quality education. Anyway, owning a diploma from a well-respected university doesn't mean that the doctor took full advantage of the school's faculty or libraries (after all, doctors have fraternities, too) or that he or she is responsible and conscientious now. Furthermore, some of those other framed documents on the wall—memberships in societies, hospital privileges, etc.—look impressive, but aren't that hard to get, because screening and documentation isn't extensive.

Board certification, however, can be one valid sign of a competent doctor. If a doctor is board certified, that means he or she has had to fulfill certain residency training and take examinations of some type to be qualified by peers. Some boards even require recertification after a set period of time.

How to Pick a Doctor
Who Wants to Be Your Health Partner

Twelve Fundamental Questions to Ask

You'll probably start your quest by asking your friends if they have already found their own Dr. Right. Nothing inspires confidence in a doctor more than hearing a good report from someone you like and respect. Sometimes, however, that's not possible—especially in large cities where thousands of doctors work. If you get a tip from a friend, find out why he likes that physician. But whether you follow a friend's lead or go "cold calling" on your own, you should get satisfactory answers to the following questions. Jot them down in a notebook, and take it with you to the doctor.

1

Does the doctor value your time?

In the Reception Area (Not waiting room!)

In general, you shouldn't have to wait longer than thirty minutes after your appointment time. Emergencies can throw a schedule off, but you should expect an apology and explanation when that happens. (It's also a good idea to call ahead and see if the doctor is running late.)

Ask if the doctor usually stays close to scheduled appointment times. And beware the doctor who orders five patients to converge on his office for a 2:00 p.m. appointment, like backed-up 747s over La Guardia Airport. Somebody's going to do some waiting, and it could be you.

Grumbling about tardy doctors is as American as griping about the latest postal rate increases, but don't despair. It's possible to find a doctor who values your time as much as you do. One way of doing that is to let your doctor know—the first time he keeps you waiting too long—that you are one impatient patient. Tell him firmly, but gently, that your time is too valuable to waste in the waiting room.

While you're waiting, you might think about the ultimate impatient patient story. Recently, after one patient was kept waiting for two hours, he sued the doctor for breach of oral contract. The doctor got the message to be more timely in a big way.

2
Is the staff courteous and friendly?

If the receptionist acts like a drill sergeant, barking commands from behind a frosted, bulletproof glass window, don't expect the other people behind that wall to be compassionate and caring. The office staff almost always gives an accurate forecast of how you'll be treated by the doctor. Remember that in building your health-care team, you're making a package deal for several players. You'll sometimes be seeing a nurse or a physician's assistant as well as the doctor, and you should be just as careful about choosing them.

3
Does the doctor or staff offer extras?

A good doctor will go the "extra mile" for patients. I don't have a waiting room; I have a reception area. Comfortable chairs, a good assortment of (current) reading material, and flowers help create an inviting environment. We even provide wheelchairs for those who need them.

If the receptionist acts like a drill sergeant, barking commands from behind a frosted, bulletproof glass window, don't expect the other people behind that wall to be compassionate and caring.

On your scouting mission, ask the receptionist or some other staff member if the doctor ever makes house calls. Home visits are rare these days, largely because a doctor can't carry along sophisticated equipment, but they are appropriate occasionally.

Does the practice ever provide a few days of sample medications to see if the drugs are helpful and tolerable? Does someone check your blood pressure, pulse, and weight as a basic preliminary? No matter the reason for your visit, the staff should show that they care about your overall medical condition.

4
Is the doctor available when needed?

This might sound obvious, but many people don't think to ask about office hours. Most people work weekdays, and a doctor who offers evening or Saturday hours can make things much easier for you. Likewise, think twice if the office closes at lunchtime. That's likely to be the most convenient time for you to make a call, and I can't understand why some doctors ignore that.

Bear in mind that if you call during office hours, a nurse or physician's assistant is likely to take your call. Nonetheless, if you do ask to speak to the doctor about a nonemergency—and don't hesitate to do so—you should receive a return call later that day or early the next morning. During the day, barring emergencies, my patients with appointments get first priority. But before I leave the office in the evening, I'm happy to return all necessary calls.

Also ask about after-hours arrangements. If you have to page the doctor through an answering service at night or on the weekend, how soon will he or she respond? In most cases, your call should be returned within fifteen to thirty minutes.

5
Whom does the doctor team up with for after-hours or weekend care?

Every doctor needs a little time occasionally when he can be sure the phone isn't going to ring. In a group practice, the members back each other up, so it's clear what your options will be when your doctor is off duty. For a doctor in individual practice, though, you should ask about backup. If your doctor is in the central city and his backup works in a distant suburb, you could spend unwanted time on the road.

6
Where are tests performed and how are the results relayed to you?

Are x-rays and other tests done in the office? While in-office testing is convenient, costs are usually higher. Also, who interprets the tests? Does the doctor read his own x-rays and electrocardiograms, or does he refer them to specialists (radiologists and cardiologists)? The primary-care doctor might be qualified, but specialists are almost certain to be.

Be sure that you will be informed of test results, whether positive or negative. That might be by letter (which has the advantage of giving you a written record), or by phone from the doctor or one of the staff members (especially when you're okay). Or the doctor might ask you to come back to the office. While it's a bit inconvenient, this might actually show caring on the doctor's part, since he or she will be able to gauge your response and provide reassurance face-to-face.

7

Is your spouse or partner encouraged to join you in the examining room?

Many people feel more comfortable being examined when a loved one is on hand, and you should remember that your partner worries, too. Besides, your spouse might be very helpful in supplying medical history. And, being a woman, there's a good chance she's had much more experience than you with doctors. Like everything in medicine, the choice is yours, but the staff should encourage you to make that choice.

8

Does the doctor listen well?

In the Doctor's Office

This might be the most fundamental of all the skills you're looking for. Because you're in the market for a partner—not someone who dictates care—the doctor should *want* to hear from you. He or she should let you tell your story uninterrupted for the first few minutes of the interview. Although you (the new, *assertive* you, remember) are going to be a very communicative patient, many people are reluctant to say just what's bothering them. A good doctor knows that it takes an active listener to help those people open up. That means undivided attention, no interruptions—and no impatient hand on the doorknob.

Many people feel more comfortable being examined when a loved one is on hand, and you should remember that your partner worries, too.

When you're talking—whether about your medical history or what the examination has turned up—you should be meeting as equals. And that means you should be fully dressed at all times except during direct examination. Some doctors actually have the horrible habit of having patients disrobe as soon as they enter the examination room. That's not what I'd consider a good sign.

9

Is the doctor eager to explain and educate?

A good doctor is a good teacher. A good patient—that's you—wants to know the details and understand his illness. He wants to know why he got sick and what he can do to prevent a recurrence. Your doctor should speak a language you can understand, and he should enjoy helping you understand.

What sort of informational handouts does the doctor offer? Are they supplied by pharmaceutical companies or written by the doctor or his staff? The latter at least indicates an extra effort on the doctor's part. Is the information up-to-date? A five-year-old handout might overlook much important new information.

10

Does the doctor provide "high touch" as well as "high tech"?

A good doctor hasn't forgotten that medicine, for all its amazing machinery and complex procedures, is still an art—an art that requires caring, compassion, and touching. As early as your get-acquainted visit, you'll be able to identify a compassionate physician. He or she will make eye contact—make sure you do, too—and seem genuinely concerned about your health.

11

Does the doctor take continuing medical education (CME) courses?

Medicine advances so rapidly that a physician has to read constantly and participate in post-graduate training to keep up. A good doctor attends two or three CME courses each year. Ask what your prospective partner does to maintain his state-of-the-art medical knowledge. When you ask about CME courses, you'll also get a hint of the doctor's area of specialization. Even general practitioners tend to concentrate on certain areas of medicine, and you're not looking for an obstetrician.

12

Does the doctor believe in trying the safest, least-expensive options first?

There are alternative treatments for just about every medical problem, and it often makes sense to try the least invasive ones first, although they might not be as certain of success. Here's a bellwether question: Ask a G.P. what approach he or she prefers for mildly elevated blood pressure. If the an-

Ask a G.P. what approach he or she prefers for mildly elevated blood pressure. If the answer involves first trying some mix of weight loss, salt restriction, and exercise, you're on the right track. If the first thing you hear is the name of a drug, it's time to look elsewhere.

swer involves first trying some mix of weight loss, salt restriction, and exercise, you're on the right track. If the first thing you hear is the name of a drug, it's time to look elsewhere.

Doing Your Part

Six Things to Do to Prepare for Your First Visit

If you're getting my drift, you've already guessed that carefully choosing a doctor doesn't end your responsibility in this partnership. In fact, it only starts it. But remember, although I'm asking you to get up out of your easy chair and get involved in your health care, doing it is going to make you feel good—both physically and emotionally.

Before your first visit, you need to do some preparation so you can give your new health partner all the information he or she needs to work with you for a healthier future. Here's a checklist for your homework:

1

Get copies of your medical records from other doctors you've seen.

These documents are actually your property, and you have every right to copies. In addition, if you've had x-rays, ask to borrow them so that your new physician can get some pictures of your past. This will save your doctor valuable interview time, which he or she can use to work on your *current* situation. In the future, medical records will likely be incorporated onto small cards that you can carry with you whenever you see a new doctor. Until then, it's better to bring your own records than it is to arrive unprepared.

2

Prepare a family history of illnesses. (Refer also to Step One.)

Because this topic is so important, I started the book with it. You should have a written record of what has ailed you and your relatives in the past, and you should bring it with you to the doctor's office, just as you would bring your checkbook.

3
Write down any problems you've had with medications.

These might or might not be a part of your medical record. Problems include allergies to medication, as well as side effects such as rashes, itching, difficulty in breathing, and rapid heartbeat. Be prepared to tell the doctor about your experience with medications, and ask questions about them. Many side effects can be reduced or eliminated by changing the dose or by taking the medication with food, a common recommendation. But you'll never know if you don't ask.

4
List any current health complaints and questions you might have. (Refer to Step One.)

Be as specific about your symptoms and the dates as you can. It saves time in the office, especially for those patients who seem to suffer from examining-room amnesia. Writing down your questions and concerns can help with nervousness or embarrassment. And remember, there's no such thing as a stupid question.

5
If you're having tests done, find out if you need to fast before your appointment.

Some tests need to be done after a night without food or, in some cases, drink. You should get explicit instructions before your appointment, preferably in writing.

6
Call ahead to see if you can provide a blood sample, or fill out forms in advance.

If you stop by the office to give a blood sample a few days before your appointment, the results should be available during your evaluation. The doctor will then be able to interpret them for you on the spot and apply that information should problems be diagnosed during the physical. Filling out the forms at your leisure means you're likely to be more thorough, and it will also help the doctor's staff get a head start on filing your insurance.

When You Need a Specialist

Even with the best health partnership, you're going to get sick now and then. Most of the time, your primary-care physician (personal/family doctor) should be able to handle your problems. For some more complicated or unusual conditions, though, you need a specialist—someone who has specific knowledge and experience with what's ailing *you*.

Medicine has advanced at such an amazing rate in the last fifty years that it's simply impossible for any one doctor to be well versed in all its aspects. To put it in concrete terms, I've learned about 90 percent of what I do in my medical practice since I finished my residency in 1979. My specialty is urology—the urinary tract, including the male genitals—and I spend several weeks each year attending conferences and continuing education courses to stay abreast of my own field. It would be a full-time job—with no time left for patients—for any doctor to keep up with all the specialties in such detail.

A specialist, in effect, knows more about less. While a general practitioner has to divide his or her energies between many different health problems, a specialist concentrates on a few. You want the doctor who has the most experience with your problem, because physician experience is one of the single most important predictors of treatment success.

Your primary-care physician often takes the lead in referring you to a specialist. But if your condition isn't improving, don't hesitate to ask for a referral.

Your primary-care physician often takes the lead in referring you to a specialist. But if your condition isn't improving, don't hesitate to ask for a referral. Never accept the explanation that there's nothing that can be done. Options always exist. If the treatment you're getting isn't working, it's time to try another. And one more thing: You need a referral any time your doctor says something like, "Well, I've never seen anything quite like this, but we can try . . . ." A good primary-care doctor knows when he's out of his league, and he shouldn't mistake you for a guinea pig.

Keep in mind that you're not just the baton being passed from one runner to another. You're a key member of the health-care team—the manager, in fact—and you need to know why you're being referred to another doctor. So be sure that your primary-care physician explains several things to you

Ask your doctor whether your records will be sent to the specialist in advance so he or she will have time to look over your case before seeing you.

in detail, including the examination or test results that led to the referral and what sort of treatment options the specialist might suggest.

Ask your doctor whether your records will be sent to the specialist in advance so he or she will have time to look over your case before seeing you. Or you might, in some cases, want to bring the records yourself. Just make sure they get there. In fact, I suggest calling before the appointment to make sure that the specialist has everything he or she needs. As a specialist, I can't emphasize too much how frustrating and fruitless it is to see a patient and not have the information I need to make a diagnosis.

Once you've been referred to a specialist, how do you know you're in good hands? If you've established a good health-care partnership with your primary-care physician, you can probably have faith in his referral; a good doctor usually can recognize another one. In addition, you might be able to get feedback from other patients who've seen the specialist. But you still need to apply the twelve questions listed earlier in this step under "How to Pick a Doctor Who Wants to Be Your Health Partner."

A good specialist stays in contact with your primary-care physician and knows when it's time to return you to home base. Once you've seen the specialist, he or she will usually send a letter to the primary-care physician describing what was found and treated. You ought to ask for a copy of that letter for your medical history. Also, ask when you should next see your primary-care doctor, and call before that visit to be sure the specialist's letter has arrived.

It's not a matter of "second-guessing" your doctor. It's a matter of doubling your chances of getting the right treatment.

Second Opinions

When should you get a second opinion? That's simple—any time your doctor recommends surgery or any other risky or very expensive procedure. It's not a matter of "second-guessing" your doctor. It's a matter of dou-

Types of Specialists and What You See Them For	
Allergist	• diagnosis and treatment of allergies
Anesthesiologist	• sedation for surgery and treatment of chronic pain
Cardiologist	• heart disorders
Dermatologist	• skin problems
Endocrinologist	• hormonal problems
Gastroenterologist	• digestive tract problems
Hematologist	• blood disorders
Internist	• specialist in adult internal organs
Oncologist	• cancer diagnosis and treatment
Orthopedist	• bone, muscle, and joint disorders
Otolaryngologist (ENT)	• ear, nose, and throat problems
Pneumonologist	• lung disorders
Proctologist	• problems with colon, rectum, or anus
Radiologist	• diagnosis with x-rays
Rheumatologist	• diseases of the joints, bones, and muscles
Surgeons	• specific areas or types of surgery
Urologist	• kidney disease, urinary tract problems including cancer, potency, male fertility

bling your chances of getting the right treatment. Any conscientious doctor will be relieved to have his or her conclusions confirmed or questioned, because that dialogue between professionals is in the best interest of the patient. On the other hand, if your doctor resists a second opinion or seems offended that another doctor disagrees, you need a new health partner. Don't hesitate to stand up for your rights. It's not just the principle; it's your health.

But if I convince you of nothing else in this book, I hope you see that *you* can and should act as a second opinion. Take advantage of all opportunities to learn about your health problem, and don't hesitate to question. In the end, no matter how many doctors you consult about what should be done, you make the final decision about treatment.

I once saw a sixty-three-year-old man who had had problems with his urination for a couple of years. He was having trouble starting, and was dribbling some. A urologist appropriately examined his prostate, did some blood work on him, and looked at his bladder with an instrument called a cystoscope.

He was told that his prostate was enlarged and he needed an operation. Naturally, that worried him, so he wanted a second opinion. He had heard me talking on the radio so he came to see me. He brought all his information with him, so I didn't have to repeat the blood test or the look into the bladder. I concurred that he had a problem with his prostate, but we discussed the fact that there were multiple options for his problem, each option having its advantages and disadvantages.

I looked at it like this: He wasn't damaging his body in any way. So it became a balancing act: How badly did the symptoms bother him, and how far was he willing to go to get rid of them?

- Option one was to do nothing, in what's called watchful waiting—just live with the symptoms and recognize that they would probably get worse with time.

- Option two was medicine that would treat the enlarged prostate either by relaxing the muscle fibers or shrinking the glandular tissue.

- Option three was the operation, a standard technique which has been around for many years, but which meant several days in the hospital and being out of commission for four to six weeks. Beyond that, there was the possibility that he might lose control of his urine and become incontinent.

- Another option was one of the newer techniques with lasers.

We discussed the advantages and disadvantages of each, and he elected to try a medication—not to cure him, but to control the problem. That medicine had some side effects we had talked about, so we tried a different one at a lower dose and that worked well for him. He's on the medication, doing fine. He's quite happy that he got a second opinion.

Second opinions are also valuable when older men have prostate cancer. There is a saying that goes, "Will a man die *from* prostate cancer or *with* prostate cancer?" That's certainly an important question as men get into their seventies and eighties, because statistics show that about 50 percent of men who die in their eighties have prostate cancer at the time of death. The real key is to predict just which men will have their lives shortened or have their quality of life affected by the cancer, which is very slow-growing.

For men in their fifties and sixties, there's no question that most of them need to have something done. Naturally, when you tell a man he has cancer, he panics and rushes right out to start talking about getting rid of it. Unfortunately, many men end up getting an operation on their prostate, which can lead to problems with erections and, more importantly, urinary control.

I know an eighty-two-year-old man who had a radical prostate surgery for cancer. He's cured of his cancer, but he's homebound now because he can't control his urine. Is he better off? Certainly not. Most urologists would not operate on a man in his eighties, and he would have been better off had he seen someone who would have presented all the options and urged him not to have the surgery.

Taking Charge

Now that you know that this health partnership is a two-way street and you're in the driver's seat, it should come as no surprise that your part of the deal doesn't stop when you walk out the doctor's door.

Now that you know that this health partnership is a two-way street and you're in the driver's seat, it should come as no surprise that your part of the deal doesn't stop when you walk out the doctor's door. To get the most from the arrangement—in fact, for it to work at all—you have to live your active role as a healthy person every day. It's really quite a good assignment. Not only will you come out healthier and wealthier, but you'll also have control over your health. When you understand what's happening to you and what can be done, fear fades away. Just carry these principles with you each day:

1

Educate yourself.

Actually, you're already doing so by reading this book. But there's much more to learn. Luckily for us, there are lots of people who want to help. Nearly every step of this book includes sources for getting more information: toll-free lines, organizations, support groups, and computer databases. Ask for and study handouts you get at the doctor's office, and research referrals yourself. You might not feel comfortable reading jargon-filled medical journals, but you don't have to: Newspapers and magazines have made great strides in covering medical developments—some of which your doctor might not know about. Tear those articles out and save them. I do, and I learn from them. Get curious and learn more about your health.

2

Ask questions.

Use what you learn to ask questions of your doctor. No good doctor minds taking the time to answer questions from a patient who's truly interested in understanding what's happening to him. Let your doctor know you want the details. Doctors aren't offended when a patient cares enough to probe—we're delighted. Once again, there's no such thing as a stupid question.

3

Get and give the whole story.

Detectives will tell you that sometimes, that little tidbit of information that seems insignificant to a witness might turn out to crack the case. Likewise, some "minor" symptom or sensation might turn out to be a key to your good health. Keep a health file—including your own copies of your medical records—and look deeply into your family medical history.

4

Tell your doctor and loved ones how you feel.

Macho, stoic attitudes do not cure diseases. If you don't tell your doctor you're in pain, he won't know to treat your pain. Likewise, express your emotions. If you're scared, say so. There's nothing wrong with being afraid of a life-threatening illness. It makes perfect sense to have fear, and men have just as much right to fear as women.

Consider how your spouse and other family members feel, too. They will often imagine you feel much worse than you do—unless you keep them informed. Women often tell me that they think their husband's disease was harder on them. A little communication is all it takes for everyone to feel much better.

5

Talk to other men about your health.

Many doctors have a list of patients who are more than willing to talk to other men about their experiences. Knowing that other guys have been in your shoes and gotten through just fine can do wonders. Us Too, the national prostate cancer support group, is one example of men helping men, and there are similar groups for impotence, heart conditions, and so forth. Ask your doctor.

Many of my patients tell me that helping others get through a problem they've experienced is the final step in their own healing.

When you graduate from your illness, you can pass the favor that someone did for you on to other men. We're in this together, and help can come from all sorts of directions. In fact, many of my patients tell me that helping others get through a problem they've experienced is the final step in their own healing. Think of it as a sort of pyramid scheme that works—and it's perfectly legal.

6

Practice what you learn.

Read the rest of this book and anything else that empowers you as a guardian of your own health. Talk to your doctor about healthful habits. Then do it! Live like your health matters, and you'll discover what healthy men know: Life isn't full or joyful until you're the master of your own fate.

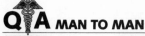

Q&A MAN TO MAN

QUESTION	ANSWER
My company's insurance coverage limits my choices for a primary-care physician, but I still want to be thorough in my search for a health partner. Any suggestions?	Even under an HMO or other plan, you still have patient rights. In Step Two, which you have just read, we gave you guidelines as to what you should expect from your health-care partner. In the next step, we explain what should be included as part of your basic care. If the assigned doctor is not living up to your standards—and your informed, assertive discussion yields no satisfaction—go to the medical director for your insurance carrier, with documented reasons in hand, and demand a change.

QUESTION	ANSWER
Whenever I call to speak to my doctor, I'm forced to talk with his nurse instead. I know she's trying to protect his time, but my time is valuable, too. Am I being treated like a second-class citizen by being denied direct contact with my doctor? After all, *he* is the one I'm paying.	Doctors certainly are busy, and it's very difficult to be interrupted during the day for nonemergencies. It's not that you aren't important—but doctors want to be fair to the patients who have scheduled appointments. In addition, nurses or other medical assistants can often answer questions or help with your needs. Still, if you don't feel you're getting what you need, insist on speaking to the doctor. Understand, though, that the conversation might have to take place at the end of the day or before normal business hours in the morning, and it might be necessary for you to speak to a staff member beforehand. That way, the staff member can gather information from you to ensure that the time spent on the phone with your physician is quality time. However, remember that no good doctor tries to diagnose over the phone. Frequently, the best solution is to come in for a face-to-face.

QUESTION	ANSWER
How can I convince a physician I've never met to give me fifteen minutes of his time for a "health-partner-ship interview?" I would think his time is too precious.	Well, let's not get hung up on exactly fifteen minutes. That's not practical, but a two- or three-minute interview shouldn't be that hard to arrange. Also, discussions with the medical and office staff can give you a good idea whether the doctor is Dr. Right for you.

QUESTION	ANSWER
What should I do if I find a primary-care physician who is perfect for me—but fails the test when I ask about back-up care?	The chances of needing a back-up depend on your medical condition. Many patients see a particular doctor for many years without ever meeting his stand-in. However, if you have a number of medical problems that increase your likelihood of having to deal with back-up physicians, you might have to consider a change.

QUESTION	ANSWER
I want to use the questions listed earlier in this step when I go seeking out a doctor, but is it okay for me to walk in holding this list in my hand? I'm not much on memoriz-ing, yet I don't want to offend the physician.	That's just fine. Don't rely on your memory. Bring the list. I'm always impressed by a patient who brings a list. Sometimes, I'll even ask to look at the list of questions to make sure I cover all of them in my discussion. A list lets me know you are involved in your care and ready to learn.

QUESTION	ANSWER
I know you're trying to be helpful, but if I do everything you recommend in this step for scouting out a primary-care physician, it could turn into a temporary part-time job. Are there any shortcuts?	I won't kid you. It's going to take some time to scout out the right physician. You might have to set priorities regarding my suggestions and decide which are the most important. That said, you might be willing to forgive a less-than-congenial receptionist. If the doctor is friendly and eager to work with you, you might overlook his being a few minutes late. Think of these as guidelines, not rigid rules.

HOTLINES	
American Board of Medical Specialists	• **(800) 776-2378**
American Institute for Preventive Medicine	• **(800) 345-2476**
Joint Commission on Accreditation of Healthcare Organizations	• **(708) 916-5800**
National Drug Information and Referral	• **(800) 662-4357**
National Second Surgical Opinion	• **(800) 638-6833**

3

**Understanding
How Medical
Tests and
Physical Exams
Can Save Your
Life**

GET PHYSICAL

MEN TALK: Willie Stevens, age fifty-seven

I went to the screening mainly because it was free. My company had a medical team in to check us men for prostate cancer, and I've never been one to turn down something for nothing.

"We had two tests. The first one was simple enough. They took a sample of blood and sent it off to be analyzed for something called PSA—prostate specific antigen. The doctor explained that it would show whether I had any prostate problems—including prostate cancer. I told him I didn't, but he said we might as well check anyway, since it was free.

"The second test involved the doctor inspecting my prostate with a gloved finger through my rectum. I have to tell you, I didn't care for it much, but it was over pretty quickly. The doctor said my prostate felt normal, and they sent me on my way—saying the blood test results would be ready in about a week.

"Six days later, I got a call saying I needed to come in for an office visit so they could repeat the blood test. To make a long story shorter, the second test confirmed the first one: My PSA was up and I needed more tests to determine if I had prostate cancer. I told the doctor it couldn't be. I felt just fine. And he told me that was good. It meant that if I did have prostate cancer, it wasn't far along and it could be cured without too much trouble.

"An ultrasound examination and biopsy confirmed my cancer, and I had an open prostatectomy—prostate removal—two weeks later. It went fine. I was out of the hospital in four days, and back on my feet in ten. It's been six months now, and everything's working pretty well. My PSA is staying down, so the cancer doesn't seem to be coming back, and I am getting back to a normal bathroom and bedroom life.

"Without that test, I wouldn't have known for a long time—maybe too long. And you know what's funny? When I went to that bulletin board to sign up, there were two sheets. One was for a baseball game, and one was for the tests. There were about a dozen men who had signed up for the cancer screening, and fifty or a hundred who had signed up for the game. I'm sure glad I made the right choice."

The First Visit: What to Expect

Once you've chosen a primary physician as your health partner, you'll want a thorough health evaluation. Even if you don't have any noticeable problems, you need a health history and physical exam for two reasons.

First, there are many medical problems that you won't notice until they're very advanced—and therefore harder to cure. And at worst, there are diseases—specifically male diseases—that are as good as death warrants by the time you detect even the first symptoms.

Second, you need an evaluation to establish a baseline. Many medical problems can be detected by charting *changes* in medical tests. Again, there might be no symptoms that you'd notice. But if the levels of some substance in your blood go up over time, it could be a life-saving early warning.

This is a key point that many people—especially men—seem to have a hard time grasping. Medical tests detect problems, but these are problems you *want* to know you have. Remember our car? You *want* to know that the brake pads have gotten so thin that they're about to grind metal against metal. That's much better than actually hearing that expensive sound. That's why it's truly good news if your physician—not you—discovers you have a disease. It means you're going to get well sooner, suffer less pain, and spend less money. These tests can be like the two-minute warning in football—a signal that it's time to hustle and make it happen before time runs out.

Organizations such as the American Cancer Society and the America Academy of Family Practitioners set guidelines for what should be done in a regular physical and how often. A group of family practitioners I work quite closely with has designed a chart utilizing these recommendations. That chart follows at the end of this step. *Bear in mind, though, that different tests are done depending on your age, family history, and other risk factors.* What's more, there are often age ranges, not exact deadlines, for performing tests. But if you wonder whether you should be having a test, ask. Never hesitate to ask why or why not.

> *That's why it's truly good news if your physician—not you—discovers you have a disease. It means you're going to get well sooner, suffer less pain, and spend less money.*

Your Health History

Building a Body of Knowledge

Your doctor should begin the physical by asking a number of questions concerning your health background, such as:

- health problems you've had in the past, going back to childhood

- diseases and health problems that run in your family

- tests and vaccinations you've had

- medications you're taking

- allergies or other problems with medications

- whether you smoke or drink

- talking about your sex life

- anything else that's troubling you now

Likewise, you should expect to be asked how things have been going—whether you feel happy and optimistic. Your health-care partner isn't just a technician; he or she is an ally and confidante.

Much of this territory can be covered on a questionnaire you fill out in the waiting room. Or, if you do the "homework" we discussed in the last step (and not while you watch a ballgame!) you can save both of you a great deal of valuable time by presenting your family history.

I can't emphasize too much that talk is vital to a good health evaluation. Your doctor needs to be an ace at getting you to voice your complaints—and not all of them are strictly physical. So don't be surprised if he or she asks some pretty personal questions—about your sex life, for instance. Many men hate volunteering information about sexual problems, though problems in bed can be emotionally devastating and can be a symptom of real physical problems that threaten your life. Too often, men don't volunteer and doctors don't make it easier by asking.

Why are these questions so important? Consider that a 1991 AMA/Gallup poll showed that more than half of those men who have experienced sexual dysfunction do not talk about the problem with their doctors. Even more alarming, four in ten doctors reported their fears that more than half of older men do not get treatment, or wait too long for treatment, of prostate cancer or colorectal cancer. Why don't they get help? Because they are reluctant to talk with their doctors about these sensitive issues.

So doctors must ask these questions. Likewise, you should expect to be asked how things have been going—whether you feel happy and optimistic. Your health-care partner isn't just a technician; he or she is an ally and confidante. You can and must be honest, and you shouldn't have the slightest doubt that your confidentiality will be respected.

Weight, Pulse, and Blood Pressure

At most doctors' offices, a nurse will weigh you, and check your pulse and blood pressure before you see the doctor. The numbers go in your file, so the doctor can look for changes from one visit to the next. Those curious over-and-under numbers, as we will soon see in a chart later in this step, can be extremely important. So if the nurse doesn't volunteer the results of these measurements, be sure to ask for them.

Weight

We are a nation obsessed with thinness, but you don't have to have basketball superstar Michael Jordan's physique to be healthy. Life insurance companies have developed tables based on height and build that show optimum weight ranges for a long life. Your doctor will want you to be within that range—not too heavy, not too light. (And contrary to the old saying, you *can* be too thin.) People who are obese—generally considered to be those who weigh more than 25 percent over their desirable weight—are much more likely to get diabetes, heart disease, and several cancers. Packing too much paunch is the number-one risk factor for high blood pressure. One study has shown a risk elevation of four and a half times above normal for overweight men.

TAKE ACTION

If you fall outside the range shown in the chart below (developed by Metropolitan Life Insurance Company), talk to your doctor about ways to lose. The next step of this book focuses on helping you shed fat.

Desirable Weight in Pounds According to Frame (dressed, with shoes on)			
HEIGHT	**FRAME**		
Feet/Inches	Small	Medium	Large
5/2	116-125	124-133	131-142
5/3	119-128	127-136	133-144
5/4	122-132	130-140	137-144
5/5	126-136	134-144	141-153
5/6	129-139	137-147	145-157
5/7	133-143	141-151	149-162
5/8	136-147	145-156	153-166
5/9	140-151	149-160	157-170
5/10	144-155	153-164	161-175
5/11	148-159	157-168	165-180
6/0	152-164	161-173	169-185

Desirable Weight in Pounds According to Frame (dressed, with shoes on)		
HEIGHT	**FRAME**		
Feet/Inches	Small	Medium	Large
6/1	157-169	166-178	174-190
6/2	163-175	171-184	179-196
6/3	168-180	176-189	184-202

Pulse

Your pulse will probably be taken at the same time as your blood pressure. A very rapid, slow, or irregular heartbeat can signal heart-rhythm problems that need correcting. Certain kinds of heartbeat irregularities might lead to heart attacks and strokes, which are life-threatening events that can be prevented by medication that stabilizes your heartbeat.

Your resting heart rate is also a good overall indicator of your physical condition. Many men find just visiting a doctor stressful enough to elevate their pulse, so they don't get an accurate measure of their resting heart rate. Try taking your own first thing in the morning before you get out of bed, as we discussed in Step One. Just count pulses for fifteen seconds, then multiply by four. Normal is around seventy beats per minute, but lower rates down to about fifty show that your circulatory system works very efficiently. Extremely low pulse rates, however, can also be a problem.

TAKE ACTION *Very rapid heartbeat—over one hundred per minute—can be controlled with medication. But if your resting pulse is even slightly elevated—over seventy-five—you should improve your level of fitness to give your heart a rest.*

Blood Pressure

High blood pressure is one of the most common and most destructive diseases—a terrible pity, because in most cases it's preventable. The American Heart Association (AHA) says that more than sixty-three million Americans have high blood pressure, yet because it has no noticeable symptoms, only half of those Americans afflicted know they're in trouble. You can't fix what you don't know is wrong.

High blood pressure puts a strain on your heart and blood vessels. It's as if some-one crimped the pipes in your home's plumbing, and the pump had to work harder to force water through the pipes.

High blood pressure puts a strain on your heart and blood vessels. It's as if someone crimped the pipes in your home's plumbing and the pump had to work harder to force water through the pipes. The pipes and pump are stressed—in the worst case, one could rupture—and not enough water might get where you want it. If your blood pressure is steadily high for extended periods, your risk of heart disease, stroke, and kidney problems shoots up.

That's why monitoring your blood pressure is vital. If you're doing it yourself, be sure to refer to the pertinent material in Step One.

Once you've got your numbers, which one is important to you? Both, as you can see from this new classification system:

Classification of Blood Pressure for Adults (Age 18 Years and Older)
(Joint National Committee of the National Institutes of Health)

Category	Systolic (mm Hg)	Diastolic (mm Hg)
Normal	< 130	< 85
High normal	130-139	85-89
Hypertension STAGE 1 (Mild)	140-159	90-99
STAGE 2 (Moderate)	160-179	100-109
STAGE 3 (Severe)	180-209	110-119
STAGE 4 (Very severe)	≥ 210	≥ 120

Based on the average of two or more readings taken at each of two or more visits following an intial screening.

TAKE ACTION

If your blood pressure regularly exceeds "high normal," you and your doctor should be discussing ways to bring it down. This new classification system will probably categorize more people as having high blood pressure, because people with normal diastolic and high systolic pressures were once not thought to be at great risk.

Once again, though, knowing you have high blood pressure is power. If your pressure is above the "high normal" level, there's a chance it won't even take drugs to solve the problem. The American Heart Association recommends a simple, painless approach of diet changes and exercise as the first line of treatment for mildly elevated blood pressure. I'll tell you how to deal with it in the next step, and we'll talk more about blood-pressure control in Step Five. And if your pressure is "high normal," you can take steps to bring it back in line, although your doctor might not consider it essential. For every point you can drop your diastolic pressure, even in the normal range, your heart attack risk drops 2 to 3 percent!

The Basic Once-Over

Getting to Know You

Working from the head down, your physician will check your body thoroughly. As he or she checks skin, breasts, testicles, and penis, you should also get a review of self-tests—both their importance and how to do them. Expect your doctor to:

- check your eyes (for acuity, voids, or dark or black spots in your field of vision, damage from high blood pressure, and—if you're older—glaucoma)

- peer and whisper into your ears (for infection and hearing problems)

- inspect your tongue and gums for signs of oral cancer (your dentist should be doing this, too)

- listen to your neck (for bruits—an abnormal sound that can indicate a clogged artery)

- check your thyroid in your neck (for swelling or lumps) examine all your skin—especially your face, ears, shoulders, and the backs of your hands (for signs of skin cancer)

- listen to your chest (for heart sounds and lung congestion, crackles, or wheezes)

- massage your chest (for lumps that might suggest breast cancer)

- probe your abdomen (for liver size, kidney and spleen problems, and abnormal masses)

- massage areas in your neck, armpits, and groin (for signs of lymph node swelling)

- check your abdomen and groin (for hernia)

- examine your testicles and penis (for cancer or other abnormalities including warts or sores)

- tap your arms, knees, ankles, and toes (for reflexes) check your muscle strength (for signs of weakness) by moving your arms and legs

- prick your arms and legs (for signs of nerve damage).

This process can take a few minutes, so why not get your money's worth and ask questions? Get tips on doing your self-exams. Inquire about why the doctor does particular things. A good health partner can explain while performing routine exams. And, besides, people who enjoy their work are usually pleased to talk about it.

Rectal Exam

Beginning at age forty, every man should have a digital rectal exam (DRE) every year. I know. Ugh. But I've found that for most guys, a rectal exam is more difficult to think about than to live through. Recently, television talk-show host Gary Collins made an excellent suggestion while we were talking before going on the "Home Show." He commented that the rectal exam was the part he dreaded most about going to the doctor, and he wondered why we don't do the rectal exam first and get it over with.

I had to agree. If a man is anxious about it, there's no reason why the rectal exam can't be done first. Don't hesitate to say so if that arrangement suits you.

Your doctor will tell you to relax (easy for him to say!), because relaxing helps your anal sphincter relax, making the exam much easier. But let's face it: When you're staring at that wall, waiting for the probe to begin, you're not in a very familiar position. Some doctors are good at making conversa-

> *If a man is anxious about it, there's no reason why the rectal exam can't be done first. Don't hesitate to say so if that arrangement suits you.*

tion to help distract you during the exam, but this isn't really the time for a good joke.

What's my solution to this stressful encounter? I ask my patients to take some deep breaths. I ask them not to clench their fists or grab the table, because that only tightens things. I have found that bearing down as the finger goes in, not straining, but bearing down as if having a bowel movement, can also help some men relax.

With some men who have had hemorrhoids or previous scar tissue, or are just incredibly uptight, I might ask them to soak in a bathtub or use some type of anesthetic or lubricant cream. I have even gone so far as to prescribe a relaxant for these men and ask them to come back later for the exam.

Maybe knowing what the doctor's going to do will relieve some of your anxiety. Here's what happens:

You'll be asked to bend over a table or lie on your side with your knees pulled up toward your chest. Your doctor will insert a gloved, lubricated finger through your anus and feel your prostate for lumps, hard spots, and overall consistency. (We call this palpation.) At the same time, the doctor will examine your rectum for abnormalities and remove a small amount of stool to examine for blood (called hemoccult or fecal occult blood test), both of which check for early signs of colorectal cancer. (The doctor might also give you a kit to take a sample at home and send back.) Other problems, such as hemorrhoids, also become obvious during a DRE.

A DRE shouldn't be painful. If it hurts, say so. It's a sign that something might be wrong with you—or with the doctor's technique. I think most men feel humiliation more than anything else, because the whole process makes them feel vulnerable. But once again, there's nothing unmanly about being smart and taking care of your body. Just keep saying to yourself, "A rectal exam is the first line in detecting prostate cancer—the second leading cancer in men." Say that a few times and it will be over.

TAKE ACTION *If your doctor detects hard spots or other abnormalities of your prostate, he or she should recommend a PSA blood test and an ultrasound examination. If either test is positive, a biopsy is in order. If blood is detected in your stool, your doctor should move you right along to the next test—sigmoidoscopy.*

Sigmoidoscopy

A digital rectal exam and fecal blood test might be the first line in detecting colorectal cancer, but the second line—for guys fifty years and older—is much more effective. With a sigmoidoscope, a doctor can actually look inside your rectum and large intestine with a lighted instrument and look for polyps (growths that might signal cancer).

Compared to having an instrument inserted in your nether regions, a DRE might sound pretty good. Sigmoidoscopy isn't really so bad, though. The scope is very thin and flexible. (If a doctor comes at you with one of the old rigid instruments, it's time to say "Stop!") And consider that a recent study at the University of Wisconsin found that the risk of dying of colorectal cancer was 80 percent lower among people who'd had sigmoidoscopy even once, compared to those who had hemoccult or rectal exams alone. Then consider that colorectal cancer is the third leading cause of cancer death in men. If you're fifty and your doctor doesn't suggest sigmoidoscopy every three to five years, ask about it.

If you have risk factors for colon cancer—a family history of the disease, for instance—or signs of colon cancer, such as change in bowel habits or passing blood, your doctor might also suggest colonoscopy, an examination of the entire large intestine. Yes, ugh again. But I repeat: These exams save lives, and one of them could be yours.

TAKE ACTION *If your doctor detects polyps, he should take samples for biopsy to see if they are cancerous.*

Tuberculosis Skin Test

Only a few years ago, TB was old news, a disease from the history books much like scurvy and diphtheria. It had pretty much been eradicated from the United States. But if you read a daily paper or watch the news, you know it's back—and in a big way. Most troubling of all, the bacterium that causes it appears to have grown resistant to many traditional medications. And that makes early detection all the more important, both to prevent TB's spread and to make a cure easier.

As with nearly every disease, the chances of a full recovery from TB are much greater when we can treat it in its early stages. As TB advances, it can create a great deal of scar tissue, which can't be repaired. That's the main reason why primary physicians I work with now recommend a *mantoux* skin test every five years from age forty on.

A mantoux test is either positive or negative. If yours is positive, you should begin treatment with appropriate medication.

Electrocardiogram (EKG)

Every time a muscle contracts in your body, it emits a small electrical current like the spark from an engine. Your heart muscle is no exception. By measuring the electrical pulses that come from it, we can learn a lot about how well your ticker is working.

To do an EKG, your doctor might have small areas of your body shaved so that electrodes can be taped to your chest, arms, and legs. (Shaving provides a better contact for the electrodes.) Signals picked up can be printed out or recorded for replay. They show us how your heart muscles are working, allow us to study your heart rhythm, and reveal signs of any previous heart attacks. (You might be surprised to learn that you can have a heart attack without knowing it.)

You might be surprised to learn that you can have a heart attack without knowing it.

EKGs are often done while you exercise, in what's called a stress test, since your heart might work fine until you ask it to work *hard*. During a stress test, you'll be asked to walk on a treadmill at a gradually increasing rate and angle of incline. As the demand for oxygen in your system goes up, the EKG can detect a lack of oxygen to the heart.

There are numerous reasons to take stress tests, including problems with erections related to blood flow, high cholesterol, or a family history of heart disease.

There are numerous reasons to take stress tests, including problems with erections related to blood flow, high cholesterol, or a family history of heart disease. A stress test is particularly important if you've decided to take up exercise after years of doing one-arm potato-chip lifts on the couch in front of the TV. Nearly everyone—even people recovering from heart attacks—can benefit from exercise, but you need to know how much and what kind. A stress test will help your doctor find out.

Regular EKGs aren't necessary until you reach your fifties—and then only once every five years. This should be a health baseline for a later comparison. However, if you have two or more of the risk factors listed under "Take Action" in the ensuing section on cholesterol (page 69), you should start getting regular EKGs while in your forties. By charting the changes in your heart's action, your doctor can see trouble coming long before it becomes life-threatening. And if you have a possible heart problem, being able to compare an old EKG to a new one might prove important.

How important? Consider that when the President of the United States travels outside of Washington, D. C., a copy of his current EKG is forwarded to his destination city. That way, in case of an emergency, doctors will have access to the report. Now I know you don't travel with Secret Service agents, but you deserve the best health care just as the President does. You should have a copy of your baseline EKG and carry it with you to each health evaluation.

TAKE ACTION

When an electrocardiogram indicates a problem, you should be referred to a cardiologist. Further tests depend on the type of problem detected.

Tetanus Booster

Here's one that goes forgotten too often. Probably because you only need one every ten years, it's easy to lose track. But a good doctor will ask when your last tetanus booster was, and when you say, "Gosh, it seems like a few years ago, but I can't remember," he or she will suggest you have one. Although tetanus (lock jaw) is rare these days, it's worth remembering that inoculation is the reason why. One of the merits of finding (and seeing!) a steady primary-care physician is that your records will be there to say for certain what you need and when.

Urine Test

A sample of urine gives a good idea of how well a significant part of your body's waste-processing system works, and also sheds light on other bodily functions. We test your urine for kidney function (protein, acidity, and concentration), infection (nitrates), diabetes (sugar), cancer and kidney stones (blood), liver function (bilirubin), and other factors. All these things are important in eliminating the possibility of serious, although uncommon, diseases, but one thing we often find out is that you're not drinking enough water (few people do). You should be drinking eight to ten glasses (eight ounces each) per day. Most of the time, you can get results of a urine test at the end of your office visit.

TAKE ACTION   *You might have blood in your urine even if you can't see it. If microscopic analysis reveals that you do, you should be evaluated with x-rays and referred to a urologist.*

Blood Tests

Most doctors offer a standard panel of blood tests (often called SMA-20) that checks cholesterol, glucose, kidney and liver function, electrolytes, and more.

Blood testing is important because it can warn us years, even decades, before a serious health problem develops. In many cases, simple changes in diet and exercise can help head off those problems. In other cases, a blood test might be the difference between life and death.

TAKE ACTION   *Many blood tests are better done while you're fasting, and most blood tests take some time to analyze. Unless you arrange to have the sample taken before your physical, results will be delayed at least* several *days and will be relayed to you by phone or a return visit.*

Cholesterol

What we commonly call a full cholesterol test is more accurately called a lipid profile, because it tells us much more than just your cholesterol level. In addition to total cholesterol, we'll find out how much low-density lipoprotein (LDL) cholesterol, high-density lipoprotein (HDL) cholesterol, and triglycerides your blood is carrying around.

- **LDL is often called "bad" cholesterol, because it's the type that forms plaque on artery walls.**

- **HDL, "good" cholesterol, appears to combat the accumulation of plaque.**

- **Triglycerides account for about 95 percent of the fats stored in your body. Although triglycerides alone don't appear to be very dangerous, recent research has shown that when both triglycerides and cholesterol are elevated, risk of heart disease goes up significantly.**

You begin to see why a simple total cholesterol measurement might not be the most accurate predictor of heart attack risk. If you have high total cholesterol, and low HDL and high triglycerides, it might indicate high risk. But if your HDL level is high—boosting the total cholesterol number—and triglycerides are normal, the risk might not be great. That's why we want to know all three.

Although I know you've heard it before, I can't overemphasize how important it is for men to watch their cholesterol levels. I don't believe in scare tactics, but here's an experience that sticks in my mind.

After we draw the blood, we place it in a centrifuge and spin it. That causes the blood cells to drop to the bottom, so what is left is the serum, which is normally clear and yellowish. But some men have such high cholesterol and triglycerides that the serum is thick like cream. On many occasions I've told these guys, "You're pumping cream through your body."

Keep in mind, too, that cholesterol problems can be affairs of the heart in more ways than one. Typically, 25 percent of the impotent men we see at the Male Health Center in Dallas have elevated cholesterol, but are unaware of it. I've told more than one man, "I can get you erections, but you might not be around to enjoy them."

TAKE ACTION

Your maximum permissible cholesterol levels are determined by your risk factors. These include:

- being a male forty-five and over
- family history of heart disease before age fifty-five
- current cigarette smoking
- high blood pressure
- HDL lower than thirty-five
- diabetes
- history of stroke or arterial disease
- obesity

If you have only male sex going against you, your total cholesterol should be less than 240 and LDL less than 160. For those of you with two or more, total cholesterol should be less than 200 and LDL less than 130. The NIH (National Institutes of Health) also says if you have definite heart disease, your LDL should be less than 100. HDL should be at least thirty-five, with the normal range running all the way up to sixty-five. With HDL, more is better.

PSA

Prostate specific antigen is produced exclusively by the prostate gland, so it's a sensitive marker for prostate cancer and other prostate troubles. Prostate cancer killed an estimated thirty-four thousand men in 1992 and can be cured only when detected early.

If you are between fifty (or forty, if you have risk factors such as a family history of prostate cancer or being African-American) and seventy years old, your blood should be analyzed for PSA every year. In general, if your PSA is higher than 4.0, something is wrong. The problem, however, could be enlargement, infection, or cancer. Repeat measurements and confirmation with other tests are necessary to diagnose any prostate problem discovered with PSA. For example, a PSA that rises slowly over the years, forming roughly a straight line on a graph, probably just shows that you're growing older and having some enlargement. If it were to curve upward, however, I'd suspect cancer.

There is certainly some controversy surrounding the PSA test. The American Urological Association and the American Cancer Society recommend that the test be done on all men at age fifty. The National Institutes of Health has not done so. There's a lack of unanimity because, as we noted in the last step, a man in his seventies might have a rising PSA level, but never be bothered by prostate cancer. Simply diagnosing cancer does not mean it has to be treated. In general, however, the more information you have the better you can make decisions.

We also use PSA to follow up on men who've had prostate removal. If we managed to get all the prostate tissue during surgery, PSA should stay close to zero. If it rises, we worry that some was missed and has begun to grow again.

TAKE ACTION *For different age ranges, different levels of PSA are appropriate. But any PSA measurement over 4.0 should be investigated further. About 25 percent of men with readings between 4.0 and ten turn out to have prostate cancer. Above ten, the odds of cancer rise sharply. I've tested men with PSA levels in the thousands.*

Blood Sugar

Glucose is the primary source of energy for bodily functions, and its level in the blood should be strictly regulated by hormones, such as insulin and glucagon. A serum glucose measurement will indicate whether diabetes or another carbohydrate metabolism problem is present.

Glucose levels below sixty or above 115 should be evaluated further with a glucose tolerance test.

In one simple test, you're tested two hours after eating, at which time your sugar levels should have returned to normal.

Other Blood Tests

The same sample of blood that tells us about your cholesterol, PSA, and blood sugar also goes through a battery of other, more exotic tests. Here's a brief rundown on what you might see on your lab analysis report:

BUN/Creatinine

Tests kidney function—detects either a basic kidney problem or blockage.

Uric acid

A result of protein breakdown, high levels can indicate kidney problems and gout.

Minerals (calcium, potassium, sodium, chloride)

Can be increased by diseases or medications; mainly, we're looking for abrupt changes.

CBC (hematocrit, hemoglobin, white blood cell count)

Can reveal infections, anemia, chronic illnesses, ulcers, leukemia, and cancer, especially cancer of the bowel.

Chest X-Ray

Chest x-rays aren't a standard part of a physical, but they can be very helpful in diagnosing heart enlargement or fluid buildup in the lungs, which can be a sign not only of lung problems but heart problems. Most of the time, though, there's one reason for giving a chest x-ray to a man—lung cancer.

Are you a smoker? I won't launch into a lecture here about why you ought to quit—I'll do that later—but I strongly suggest that you have a regular chest x-ray if you insist on smoking, or if you quit only recently. Although lung cancer is one of the most frustrating cancers to cure, medical science is making progress. Just in the last year, pioneering techniques have been developed for removing small lung cancers without cutting you wide open. But I emphasize: *small* cancers. If the cancer gets too large, there's not much we can do.

Your doctor ought to recommend a chest x-ray if you smoke, and even more important, he should be

Suggested Guidelines for Regular Examinations and Preventative Measures for Men					
PROCEDURE	INTERVAL	AGE			
		20-29	30-39	40-49	50+
Physical Exam	Every 3 years	X	X		
	Every 2 years			X	
	Every year				X
Blood Pressure	Every year	X	X	X	X
Tuberculosis	Every 5 years	X	X		
Blood and	Every 3 years	X	X		
Urine tests	Every 2 years			X	
	Every year				X
Electrocardiogram	Every 3-5 years				X
	Every 3-5 years (high risk)		X		
Tetanus booster	Every 10 years	X	X	X	X
Rectal exam	Every year			X	X
PSA Blood Test	Every year				X
Hemoccult	Every year			X	X
Sigmoidoscopy	Every 3-4 years				X
Chest x-ray	Every year (if a smoker)		X	X	

Note: Intervals and frequencies might vary depending on factors such as family history and your smoking habits. (Developed by Richard Honaker, M.D., and Family Medical Association of Texas, P.A., 1993)

working with you to help you quit. Research increasingly shows that many of the problems caused by smoking can be reversed if you stop. It's the single most important act in preventive medicine.

Depending on what the x-ray detects, you should be referred to a cardiologist, pulmonologist, or oncologist.

Making Sense of It All

Once the actual examination is finished, you should get dressed and sit down for a talk with your doctor. Start by asking any (and all!) questions that have occurred to you. Any question is a good question. The doctor should thoroughly describe what he or she looked for and found. If you have any specific health problems, they should be described in language you can understand, and the physician should offer several options for treating them.

If there's something you need to do by way of diet or other behavioral changes, don't trust your memory. Ask for written instructions. If you're to receive a medication, ask about side effects and whether you should be taking it at particular times (with or after meals, for example). If further tests are called for, ask about scheduling. Could you have them on a Saturday at a hospital, for example? Do you need to prepare (by avoiding food, for example)?

A good physician includes you in your health-care plan. Remember, too, that your doctor is an educator. Ask about the latest information on risks, warning signs and symptoms, tests, and treatment options. Your interest in the details will tell your doctor that you really care.

Ask for a copy of the examination and test results as well as the summary letter the doctor will prepare for your file, so you can add these documents to your medical history file.

All this information can be a little overwhelming. If you like, tell your doctor you're going to take the results home, sort things out at your leisure, and come back later to ask questions. Remember, you're starting an ongoing dialogue with your health-care partner.

If you have any specific health problems, they should be described in language you can understand, and the physician should offer several options for treating them.

MAN TO MAN

QUESTION	ANSWER
I read that some doctors think a vasectomy might cause prostate cancer. Should I start having prostate exams sooner if I've had a vasectomy?	Some studies show a link between vasectomy and prostate cancer. Of course, others don't. At this point, there's no solid proof—I'll talk about this in more detail in a later step—but it's still wise to take the careful approach. If you had a vasectomy twenty or more years ago and are still under fifty, I recommend that you start having PSA tests each year. Of course, you've been having your annual digital rectal exam, right?

QUESTION	ANSWER
My father and grandfather both had strokes, and I have mildly elevated blood pressure. My doctor wants me to have a blood test each year for red-blood-cell count (among other things). Why?	Red blood cells affect the viscosity of your blood, and stroke risk is related to that thickness. By monitoring your red blood cell count, your doctor knows whether to prescribe a blood thinner to reduce your stroke risk.

QUESTION	ANSWER
I've already had a mild heart attack, and my doctor doesn't think I'm up to an exercise stress test. She recommends a chemically based stress test. What is it and is it as good?	You're one of about three-quarters of a million people each year who ought to, but can't have a stress electrocardiogram. An alternative—dipyridamole imaging—involves injecting you with the drug dipyridamole to increase blood flow by three to five times. A subsequent injection of a radioactive tracer allows a radiologist to track the blood through your system with an x-ray. Plugged vessels don't show up well on the film, indicating where you have problems. Dipyridamole imaging is approved by the Food and Drug Administration (FDA), but it's available only at larger medical centers.

QUESTION	ANSWER
For the first time, my blood pressure was up when I last visited my doctor. Should I be worried about a single high reading?	You shouldn't worry about it, but you should follow up on it. Blood pressure varies quite a bit. You could have been under a lot of stress that day—some people get high blood pressure just going to the doctor (the aforementioned "white coat syndrome")— or the reading could have shown a real change in your body. I suggest you have repeat measurements at your doctor's office. And consider monitoring your own blood pressure so you can measure it at different times during the day. The important thing isn't how high your blood pressure is at one moment. It's your average blood pressure that matters.

HOTLINES	
Agency for Health Care Policy Research	• **(800) 358-9295**
American Academy of Family Physicians	• **(800) 274-2237**
National Council on Patient Information Education	• **(202) 347-6711**
National Health Information Center	• **(800) 336-4797**
Rare Disease Hotline	• **(800) 456-3505**

4

Eating and Exercising for Better Health

FUELING AND TUNING

E very other chapter of this book starts with a personal story from one of my patients. Over the years, being a doctor has offered me the privilege of meeting many inspiring men—men who have overcome their male health problems and want to help other men avoid or overcome the same problems. I wanted those men to speak in my book, because health troubles are more than symptoms, tests, and treatments. They're things that happen to real people.

So when it came time to write about nutrition, exercise, and weight control, I pored back over my memories, looking for just the right guy to talk about how hard getting fit and staying fit is for most of us, how much easier it can be than you think, and how much it can do for you. Try as I might, though, I couldn't think of a better example than myself. So here's my story—followed by the scientifically established methods that helped me succeed. You can, too.

MEN TALK: Ken Goldberg, age forty-five

I have had trouble controlling my weight for most of my life. As a boy, I was too heavy to participate actively in most sports, and fat continued to haunt me as a man. I tried all the standard diet approaches: counting calories, gimmick diets, substitutes, protein, groups (food groups, not therapy groups), and the rest.

Most of these wonder diets just sapped my energy and made me miserable and irritable. Sometimes I wonder how my wife put up with me.

"And after all that misery, none of the diets worked. I'd lose the weight, but I always gained it back. When people ask, I tell them I've lost three hundred pounds— dropping thirty pounds at least ten different times. I know the frustration that so many men feel about losing weight.

"Not once in my younger years did I ever seriously consider exercise. The very idea of running when nothing was on fire seemed ridiculous, and I can remember laughing at a medical school roommate who worked out three times a week. Who was this clown trying to impress, anyway? I smoked a pack of unfiltered cigarettes a day—two packs when I was feeling energetic— and tried to starve off the pounds.

"My weight problem, along with the cigarettes, followed me into the first years of my medical practice. At 6-foot-1, I was lugging around 285 pounds. I can't tell you how frustrating and embarrassing it was to be a doctor—a health expert—who was overweight. What was that old line from the Bible? 'Physician, heal thyself.' As I advised some overweight man to lose weight, I sometimes felt a bit hypocritical. Was he looking at my waistline? I knew that fat could steal years from my life span, but I seemed unable to do anything lasting about it. Lucky for me, I'm blessed with a good family health history, which is probably why I developed no serious problems.

"Today, at forty-five, I'm a new man. Few people who meet me guess I ever had a weight problem, and old classmates who saw me at a recent high school reunion barely recognized me. I eat more than ever and enjoy it without guilt. Best of all, I have more energy than I've ever had in my life. I start at 5:00 a.m. and go to 10:00 p.m.

"How did this amazing transformation take place? It wasn't because I suddenly developed more willpower or thought up some revolutionary scheme. Not at all.

With the support of a very fit and caring spouse, I learned two simple truths: 1) Exercise and eating are inseparable, and 2) what you're made of is more important than how much you weigh.

"Don't get me wrong. Although I've got a handle on my problem, it's still not easy. There is a fat person inside me who feels he's been denied visitation rights, and it's a constant fight to avoid slipping back into old habits. As a nutritionist friend says, 'It's O.K. to deviate, but you've got to get right back on track.' To this day, my closet still holds two wardrobes—fat and thin—to remind me what I'll look like if I don't. But I've found an approach that does work, and I know I'll stick with it."

The Winning Combination: How Food and Exercise Work Together

Most of us understand that exercise burns up calories. Like a car, if you go slowly, you'll use less fuel. People who suffer from couch-potato syndrome tend to be overweight. But there's more to it than just how far down you push your body's gas pedal. *How* you push the pedal—your driving style—also makes a difference. By exercising in certain ways, you can encourage your body to use up your stores of fat, and you can replace that fat with muscle.

Likewise, most of us can readily understand that certain foods give us more instant energy than others. A glass of fruit juice helps shake out the cobwebs first thing in the morning, just as a heavy evening meal puts us to sleep. Once again, though, there's more to it than just picking the right grade at the pump. Have you ever noticed that in luxury cars you're told to use premium gasoline, but you don't see that warning on lower-priced cars?

Which brings us to the most important difference between a car and your body: You can always trade in your car, but you're stuck with your body. By carefully combining proper eating and exercise, you can

You can always trade in your car, but you're stuck with your body.

rev up your engine from an anemic four-cylinder into a hot V8. You'll have (and burn) more energy every moment of the day (and night)—more energy for work, for play, and, yes, for sex. But you can't do it with food or exercise alone. It takes the right mix of the two to build the muscles that will turn you into a Corvette.

Forget Diets. You Can Eat All You Want if You Eat Right.

During the 1980s, dieting became a national obsession in the United States. Dozens upon dozens of diet gurus wrote bestsellers hawking weight-loss schemes. Major national corporations were created to help people shed fat. Yet according to a Louis Harris survey, more Americans than ever are overweight: 66 percent in 1992 versus 58 percent in 1983. As you can surmise from the thousands of fast-food places that line our highways, we're a nation of blimps.

What went wrong? I think we can pin the blame on some other numbers, those on the bathroom scale. Almost without exception, people measure their success by how many pounds they've lost—although merely weighing less doesn't guarantee that you're in good shape. There's good weight and bad weight, as you can see by looking at professional athletes. Many of those guys carry a lot of weight—but you don't see much fat on those frames.

And how do people try to lose those pounds? By cutting calories. The very word "diet"—which originally meant a way of living—has come to mean nothing more than eating less—and hating it, most of the time. In the name of these diets, millions of people suffer intense hunger, eat foul-tasting concoctions, and make themselves sick from nutritional deficiencies—all to no avail, in most cases. They might lose a few pounds temporarily, but the baggage almost always comes back. Little wonder. Not only does starvation make you miserable, it doesn't work.

Why not? Because your body doesn't understand diets. The human body evolved long before there

Almost without exception, people measure their success by how many pounds they've lost—although merely weighing less doesn't guarantee that you're in good shape.

were Five-Day Miracle Munchie Diets and aging sports figures selling Slender Goo. Therefore, any sudden drop in calories is perceived as a real threat to survival. Your body doesn't know that you're just worried about getting into last year's tuxedo. For all your body knows, you're stranded near the Arctic Circle and you're down to your last chunk of seal meat.

So your body, in its wisdom, does a perfectly sensible thing: It tries to save itself by cutting the amount of energy it burns. Metabolism—the base rate at which your body uses fuel—drops significantly when you diet. That's why people often feel sluggish during diets—and it's why they regain weight after they go off the diet. When they return to something close to their normal food intake, their confused bodies can't utilize all of the new calories, and the fried chickens come home to roost. Studies show that more than 90 percent of people who lose by dieting alone regain the weight.

Worse, one of the first things to go when you cut calories is lean muscle mass. Remember, the body thinks it's in real trouble. Someone has pulled the plug. So, since muscle takes more energy to maintain than fat, the dieting body jettisons it. Fat is your life preserver, so when you starve your body, it holds on to fat until the bitter end. What an irony. By cutting calories, you end up getting the opposite of what you want: You're building a fat, low-efficiency body with a slower metabolism. The biggest loss is body fluid.

There's no need to suffer to control your weight. In fact, to lose fat and gain muscle—that's what we really want, isn't it?—you may need to eat *more*, not less. Eat the right foods and get exercise, and you can increase your calorie intake while you shed fat, in part because you're increasing your metabolism. Look at me. When I'm really exercising and eating the right foods, I can eat twenty-five hundred to three thousand calories a day.

Besides helping you lose unsightly body fat that puts you at risk of a host of male health problems, a balanced nutrition plan will protect your health in other ways. As you'll learn in the next step of this book, certain foods contain nutrients that are recognized to help prevent cancer, heart disease, and other life-threatening ailments. For now, though, let's look at the satisfying elements that make up a healthful program for a lifetime—one that will help you finally achieve what cutting calories couldn't.

A Simple Formula

I know you've heard it many times before, but have you ever thought about what the phrase "You are what you eat" actually means? It might be the single most important gem of nutritional wisdom there is. Consider the three major categories of nutrients and what they're apt to turn you into.

Fat

Eating fat tends to make you fat. For a variety of reasons, *dietary* fat is especially effective at putting *body* fat on you. First, fat packs more than twice as many calories (nine versus four per gram of food) as the other two main food forms (protein and carbohydrate). But even if you count calorie for calorie, fat outranks the competition in building a spare tire. Because your body uses less energy processing fat than the other food types, more of its energy can be stored (as fat).

Some fat is absolutely essential to good nutrition. When I have a patient in the hospital who hasn't been able to eat for ten to fourteen days because of a serious condition, he will get some intravenous free fatty acids as part of his care. But that's an extreme situation. Most people in wealthy nations eat almost four times as much fat as they really need. You actually only need about 10 percent of your calories from fat to be healthy, but the typical American man's diet is 35 to 40 percent fat. Not surprisingly, his body is composed of 25 or more percent of fat—instead of the 15 percent or less that will make him healthier and feel better.

Protein

This controversy is complicated by the fact that your minimum need for protein is related to your body size, not to the amount you eat.

Protein is what muscles are made of. Unlike fat, it contains nutrients (amino acids) that are absolutely necessary to form muscle, and it helps repair damage to your body from illness or surgery. Not only that, it requires more energy to process—meaning you can put more in without having leftover calories that are turned into body fat. Standard nutritional wisdom says that most Americans get sufficient protein (about 15 percent of calories), but the subject is controversial among nutritionists. Some argue that more protein is helpful in maintaining muscle, particularly in people who exercise intensively, while others argue that the best sources of protein—animal products—also contain fat, which should be avoided.

This controversy is complicated by the fact that your minimum need for protein is related to your body size, not to the amount you eat. So talking about percentage of calories has limited relevance. The adult male's Recommended Dietary Allowance (RDA) for protein—as established by the National Research Council, an organization that updates its RDAs every five to ten years—is about one-third of a gram per pound of body weight. So a guy who weighs 160 pounds should be getting at least fifty-three grams of protein a day. That's not much. A chicken breast and a cup of nonfat yogurt will get you there. On the other hand, levels up to almost a gram per pound (almost 160 grams per day for a 160-pound man) are generally thought not to be harmful, unless there is a kidney problem.

The sensible approach is to try a level somewhere in between—taking care to get that protein from low-fat sources such as skinless chicken or turkey, fish, and nonfat dairy products—and see how it works for you. If you're not satisfied, get some expert advice. Your doctor might be able to help, but he or she isn't necessarily well trained in nutrition. (Remember, not all medical schools offer nutrition courses.) As an alternative, look for a dietitian or clinical nutritionist—but bear in mind the things we talked about in Step Two. Ask questions of any health professional to establish credentials and to be sure the person stays up-to-date with the latest developments in the field. You're looking for someone who's more than just a calorie counter.

Carbohydrate

Carbohydrate, our third major food type, is the fuel we burn immediately to stay warm and move about. Some carbohydrate that is not immediately burned up is stored in the muscles and the liver as a substance called glycogen. That's what keeps me going on those mornings when I run three miles on nothing but a bowl of cereal. The cereal might not be enough to fuel that trip, so my heart, lungs, and muscles draw on the glycogen reserves. Our bodies can readily turn it into the materials we need to make our hearts beat, our toes tap, and our eyes see. Once the body has filled its tanks with glycogen, the excess carbohydrate is stored as fat.

Unfortunately, it's not quite as simple as shoveling down spoonfuls of sugar (a carbohydrate). Carbohydrate needs to be divided into two general classes—simple and complex—when we talk about feeling energetic and controlling obesity:

SIMPLE CARBOHYDRATE

Table sugar, for example—breaks down relatively quickly in your digestive tract, offering a burst of energy. Unfortunately, unless you're busy running a marathon, there's likely to be more energy than you need at the moment, and excess gets stored as—you guessed it— fat. A big problem with simple sugar is that it's almost addictive. Because it processes so quickly, it gives you a surge of energy. But then you crash—unless you have more sugar.

COMPLEX CARBOHYDRATE

Complex carbohydrate takes longer to be processed in your body, so it provides a steadier supply of energy. It also takes more energy to process than simple sugars, although both beat fat. For most people in most situations, complex carbohydrate works much better.

On the average, Americans get about 40 to 45 percent of their calories from carbohydrate, and a third to a half of that is in the simple form. Conventional nutritional wisdom says we ought to get 50 to 55 percent of our calories from carbohydrate, with only a small part of that in simple form.

There is, however, good reason to get substantially more of your daily energy needs from carbohydrate—in the 60- to-65-percent range—with most of it complex. If you cut your fat intake to 20 percent of calories—10 percent better than the modest goal of 30 percent set by the American Heart Association—that leaves 80 percent of your diet to divide between protein and carbohydrate. If 15 or 20 percent of that is protein, between 60 and 65 percent will be carbohydrate. A fair amount of evidence says that people who push the upper limits on carbohydrate feel better, have lower cholesterol, and live longer.

Putting Together a Dietary Plan Based on the Three Sources

Get The Fat Out

So we've established that the first principle of healthy eating is to cut the fat from your diet. Although the AHA, as we just said, recommends holding fat to less than 30 percent of total calories, you should try to keep your dietary fat below 20 percent of calories if you're serious about losing body fat. And if you have heart troubles, even less may be better. Dr. Dean Ornish of the University of California, San Francisco, has shown that a combination of very low fat diet (10 percent), exercise, and relaxation can actually reverse heart disease.

Initially, it's not easy to cut fat because our taste buds have gotten so used to it. Most Americans are conditioned to think fat tastes good. But in time, your palate changes and you get used to a lower-fat diet. In fact, in my experience—and I have lots of friends who agree—once I had been on a low-fat diet for a couple of months, fatty foods started to have a sort of disgusting, slippery texture to them.

Although the American Heart Association recommends holding fat to less than 30 percent of total calories, you should try to keep your dietary fat below 20 percent of calories if you're serious about losing body fat.

How low should you go on fat? Figuring out your exact fat intake would require crunching a bunch of numbers, but you don't really have to pack a calculator to eat. Follow a few simple guidelines, and your fat intake will automatically drop to more healthful levels.

1
Avoid red meat.

Fat Facts
The simplest way to eat less fat is to make red meat a rare visitor on your plate. In general, beef (other than veal) and pork products have the highest fat contents of all meats. Fish, turkey, and chicken are lower in fat. When you *do* eat red meat—and rules are made to be broken—trim the fat off before you cook it.

2
Avoid prepared foods.

In general, the frozen food section at the grocery store is Fat City. What sounds healthful—an Italian meal with spinach, for example—all too often turns out not to be. Additionally, Chinese food—which can be good for you—can be high in fat, too, when ordering egg rolls or fried rice. Whole milk, cheese and cream can bump fat content up to 50 percent or more. Food labels that can be deciphered by people without higher degrees in mathematics are on their way, but in the meantime, avoid foods that list more than about one-third of their calories as coming from fat. And remember, each gram of fat equals nine calories.

3
Beware of sauces.

Likewise, a creamy dressing can add half a day's worth of fat to an otherwise low-fat salad.

Fat can also slip into your diet through sauces. Cheese-based hollandaise, for example, can turn a healthful serving of broccoli or cauliflower into a fatfest. Choose low-fat alternatives—low-fat sour cream, for example—at home, and ask for sauces on the side when you dine out. Likewise, a creamy dressing can add half a day's worth of fat to an otherwise low-fat salad. When you ask for it on the side, you'll find you need to use only a small fraction of the serving to enjoy the flavor.

4
Opt for broiled, baked, or steamed foods, and avoid fried foods.

Lean food cooked in fat becomes fat food. Hash brown potatoes, for example, sound like a great low-fat alternative to deep-fat-fried potatoes—until you realize that they're grilled in fat. I like to slice a potato, season it and stick it in the broiler. Then right before it's done, I sprinkle some nonfat cheese on it. Good stuff.

5
Don't eat traditional snack foods.

Chips, nuts, and crackers are loaded with fat. If you're snacking because you're hungry, eat a balanced, small meal (protein, complex carbohydrate, and a small amount of fat). For a social snack, try vegetables (carrot sticks, celery, etc.), popcorn (no butter, but substitutes work well), or whole-wheat pretzels.

6
Eat a meatless evening meal.

Try to eat a meatless evening meal, such as pasta prima vera, or beans and rice, at least twice a week. Additionally, limit your daily intake of meat to six ounces or less.

Not All Fats Are Created Equal

It's both necessary and inevitable that you eat some fat, but what kind? Technically, there are three major types of fat: saturated, polyunsaturated, and monounsaturated. A growing body of evidence suggests that saturated fat is the bad guy when it comes to cholesterol and, perhaps, even some cancers. For example, people who eat what is called a Mediterranean diet—lots of olive oil (a monounsaturate), but little saturated fat—have unusually low rates of heart disease.

So when you do eat fat, try to make it monounsaturated or at least polyunsaturated. The accompanying list gives you some examples of the three types, but you don't even have to read labels to choose. *Just avoid fats that are solid at room temperature.* All saturated fats and a group of modified polyunsaturates called hydrogenated fats (margarine, for example) are solid at room temperature. The thicker a fat is at room temperature, the more effectively it will clog your arteries.

If you need a substitute, olive oil and canola oil are better than bacon grease.

EXAMPLES OF TYPES OF FATS		
Monounsaturated	**Polyunsaturated**	**Saturated**
Olive oil	Corn oil	Butter
Canola oil	Safflower oil	Coconut oil
Avocado oil	Sunflower oil	Palm oil

Make no mistake, though. When it comes to putting fat on your body, all fats are created equal—equally bad. If you need a substitute, olive oil and canola oil are better than bacon grease. But if you eliminate the need for oil entirely, you've done yourself a service. Remember, we want to keep our fat level low.

Eat Quality Protein

As you cut fat by reducing the amount of red meat, whole milk, and high-fat snack foods in your diet, you need to be sure you get adequate protein. While it's true that many foods high in protein are also fatty, the two are in no way connected. Don't condemn protein through guilt by association. Your body needs it to build new tissue (muscles, for example) and to support basic biological processes. Here are some examples of quality protein:

- Fish
- Turkey (skinless white meat)
- Chicken (skinless white meat)
- Veal
- Egg whites
- Skim milk and ½-percent milk
- Low-fat dairy products

All the Complex Carbohydrates You Want

In addition to our two major classes of carbohydrates—simple sugar and complex carbohydrate— we need to identify a third kind created by mankind. Since grains began to be extensively processed in the twentieth century, many complex carbohydrates have been rendered closer to simple sugars in function. White flour, for example, breaks down more quickly in your digestive tract than its whole-wheat predecessor.

EXAMPLES OF SIMPLE, PROCESSED, AND COMPLEX CARBOHYDRATES		
Simple	Processed	Complex
Sugar	White bread	Whole grains
Honey	Pasta	*(including whole wheat pastas)*
Some fruits	Bagels	Legumes *(peas, beans, etc.)*
Dairy products	Most crackers	Potatoes
Corn syrup	White rice	Oatmeal
		Brown rice

Unless your body is prepared to make use of them with intense activity, excess foods —regardless of source (sugar, starch, protein, fat, and even alcohol)—get stored as body fat. Thus, it is recommended that you:

1 Eat smaller, more frequent meals.

2 Avoid consuming a large meal in the evening.

3 Stay away from high-fat evening snacks washed down by a beer or a soft drink.

If you exercise, your body will be able to handle a certain amount of simple sugar and processed carbohydrate without too much difficulty, but you're still better off sticking to slower-burning complex carbohydrates. They'll help even out your energy level during the day—especially when combined with protein—and they're much richer in important nutrients. I'll hold the discussion of those nutrients and their disease-preventive capabilities for Step Five, but there is one constituent of complex carbohydrates that you should try to include as a general part of your nutrition plan—fiber.

Swapping Fat for Fiber

In many ways, fiber is the opposite of fat. Instead of being absolutely packed with calories, it contains almost none. Instead of making you fat, it's likely to help you lose weight. Instead of making you constipated, it promotes regularity. Instead of promoting colorectal cancer, it might help protect against it.

Fiber—in the form of whole grains, fruits, and vegetables—is a nutritional champ. Fiber does not contain vitamins and minerals, but foods high in fiber provide an abundance of many vitamins and minerals. The National Cancer Institute recommends twenty-five grams of fiber a day. As the new food labels ordered by the FDA become available, you'll be able to track your fiber intake in a detailed way. Meanwhile, just be sure you include some in your meals at least a couple of times each day.

EXAMPLES OF HIGH-FIBER FOODS		
Whole-wheat bread	Pasta	Oat bran
Brown rice	Beans	Broccoli
Cabbage	Carrots	Prunes
Apples		

Fruits and Vegetables Guys, our parents were right. The orange, yellow and green vegetables—including broccoli, carrots, and cauliflower—are a great source of vitamins and minerals. Vegetables also have very few calories (if you avoid the dressings, and stick with imitation butter and seasonings) and they're rich in antioxidants which can help ward off cancer. Try to have at least two or three servings a day of vegetables, not just with meals, but also as snacks. Okay, munching raw carrots might not seem as macho as wolfing down a deep-fried chicken leg dripping with grease, but they're filling and good for you. Maybe you'll start a new trend with your buddies. By the way, don't ignore fruits—they are a great source of vitamin C and soluble fiber.

How to Eat (Meal and Snack Planning)

How to eat? "With a knife, fork, and spoon," you might respond. But there's a simpler and more delicious answer: Eat often. Research indicates that eating the same amount of calories in frequent small meals—particularly if they're well-balanced, low-fat meals—will improve weight control and might lower your total cholesterol and LDL ("bad" cholesterol).

Get in the habit of always asking yourself why you're about to eat before you eat.

You'll be more likely to lose fat if you eat more often, and you'll be full of energy as well. I try not to go more than three hours during the day without eating something. I used to drink six or seven cups of coffee a day, but I don't need the caffeine buzz to keep me going now. At mid-morning or mid-afternoon, when I find myself beginning to slow down, I eat a little piece of baked or broiled chicken (without skin), and either rice or potato, and my energy level comes right back.

At the very least, be sure you don't miss the most important meal of the day—breakfast. In his ten-year study of Californians, Dr. Lester Breslow of the University of California at Los Angeles found that men who ate breakfast regularly and practiced other healthy habits were half as likely to be disabled or die prematurely as those who did not follow these habits.

Finally, get in the habit of always asking yourself *why* you're about to eat before you eat. Are you truly hungry, or are you about to eat because you're nervous? Far too much eating gets done for social or emotional reasons rather than real hunger.

Water: The Essence of Life

Water doesn't pack too much nutritional punch, but nothing else can take its place. With the exception of air, there is no other compound that we can get along without for a shorter time—a few days. Water makes up more than half of our bodies. Aside from being fundamental to our existence, water also happens to be the perfect natural medicine. Did you know, for example, that water:

- is a diet aid? It fills your stomach with zero calories, and it might help your body burn fat.

- is a natural laxative? It helps you digest your food and pass waste easily.

- protects your joints? Synovial fluid lubricates joints, and it increases as water intake increases.

- helps head off wrinkles? Good skin tone is dependent on elasticity, which water promotes.

- prevents kidney stones? When the kidneys don't get enough water, salts may crystallize, forming painful stones.

- cures hangovers? If you must drink, dilute the alcohol with water to relieve headache and other hangover symptoms.

- prevents urinary tract problems? A well-flushed system is less likely to be susceptible to infection.

You should be drinking at least eight to ten glasses (eight ounces each) of water every day. Keep some near you during the day and sip regularly. You'll be amazed how much better you feel.

THE DAILY LINEUP	
Carbohydrate	• 3/5 of calories
Protein	• 1/5 calories
Fat	• 1/5 of calories
Fruits	• 2-3, or more, servings
Vegetables	• 2-3, or more, servings
Water	• 8-10 glasses (approx. eight oz. each)
(NOTE: This intake of vegetables and fruits meets your daily fiber needs)	

Exercise for Health

Until a few generations ago, most people got enough exercise to keep them reasonably fit just by doing what needed to be done in a day. But since automobiles, electricity and eight-hour sitting jobs came along, exercise has gradually been removed from our everyday lives. It seems unlikely to me that the increase in obesity—not to mention the rate of heart disease—over the same period is a coincidence. A tremendous volume of scientific research shows that regular exercise promotes not only fat control, but also a healthier heart and a more energetic life. Dr. Breslow's study, for example, found that being active in sports was the most po-

A tremendous volume of scientific research shows that regular exercise promotes not only fat control, but also a healthier heart and a more energetic life.

tent way to head off an early death—more effective, even, than quitting smoking, losing weight, or giving up booze.

So if your behind is the only part of you that's been getting a workout, it's time you got up off your duff and experienced life fully. Check with your family doctor to be sure you don't have any health problems that might restrict your activity, and then establish a well-balanced fitness program. The American Heart Association has a checklist. (Refer to the end of Step Five for the telephone number.)

It's customary to divide exercise into two distinct types. One is aerobic exercise (fitness), which can be done for long periods of time, because you're utilizing large amounts of oxygen for energy production. The other type of exercise is strength training. The distinction between the two *is* important, as long as you don't make the all-too-common assumption that only aerobic exercise really matters. Both types of exercise are vitally important to your program to shed fat and get in shape.

Aerobic Awareness

Achieving and maintaining aerobic fitness is far easier and much less painful than you might imagine from watching TV workout programs. You don't need to gasp for breath or run marathons—or for that matter, run at all—to get there. In fact, that's not even desirable.

Dr. Kenneth H. Cooper, founder and director of the Cooper Aerobics Center (just down the street from the Male Health Center in Dallas, Texas), has dedicated years of careful research to determining both what aerobic exercise can do for you and also just how much you need. He's found that aerobic fitness—and the dramatic improvements in cardiovascular health that come with it—is not won through suffering. In carefully controlled research reported in the *Journal of the American Medical Association*, Dr. Cooper's associates note that a group

> *Indeed, aerobic exercise is something we can all do easily and without risk.*

of patients walking slowly (twenty minutes per mile) showed the same decrease in the risk of heart disease as a group walking much faster (twelve minutes per mile) and also showed substantial improvement in fitness.

Indeed, aerobic exercise is something we can all do easily and without risk. It's simply a matter of tuning your body to operate more efficiently by participating in an activity that raises your heart rate above normal at least thirty minutes per day, about three times per week. Yes, an hour and a half a week is all it takes.

Just this past summer (1993), the U.S. Centers for Disease Control and Prevention, and the American College of Sports Medicine reported that you can get significant aerobic benefits by "accumulating" thirty minutes or more of moderate-intensity physical activity over the course of most days of the week. Some of the cumulative activities might include walking fast to the bus stop, mowing the lawn (but not with a riding mower), and climbing the stairs at work. Take two fifteen-minute exercise breaks at work—one in the morning and one in the afternoon on days you can't get a workout of thirty or more minutes in. Such an exercise break can consist of a short, brisk walk outside.

The FIT Formula: Frequency, Intensity, Time

There's an easy acronym to remember when setting up your fitness program: FIT. Frequency, intensity, and time are the elements to consider when you're going for true fitness.

The frequency, as we just said in the previous section of aerobic awareness, should be three times a week. The time? Experts disagree as to how much needs to be done in one interval, but they agree you need to get at least thirty minutes a day.

The intensity part is a bit more complex. Some experts prefer what's known as the (Gunnar) Borg Scale of Perceived Exertion. As the words imply, this involves tuning in to your own feelings as you exercise, monitoring *how the exercise feels to you*. In effect, you're finding the limits of your endurance, then pushing your own envelope. It makes sense, if you think about it. After all, the charts and the machines aren't out there knocking out the miles. You are.

BORG SCALE OF PERCEIVED EXERTION														
6	7	8	9	10	11	12	13	14	15	16	17	18	19	20
	Very, very light		*Very light*		*Fairly light*		*Somewhat hard*		*Hard*		*Very hard*		*Very, very hard*	

The exercise intensity required to obtain fitness is located right in the middle of the Borg chart, and intensity is associated with a feeling of somewhat hard.

To give you some idea of what these terms mean, consider a very, very light case of exertion something like a slow walk in the mall. On the other hand, a very, very hard exertion would be running away from someone or some animal chasing you. You want to keep your workouts in the somewhat-hard range where you are focused on your exercise, yet are able to carry on a conversation at the same time.

Training Heart Rate

The other, equally valid way of measuring intensity is by figuring your training heart rate. Short of hooking you up to machines that actually measure all your vital signs, we can calculate a working heart-rate range based on your age and a standard of 220.

For example, if you're 42 years old, subtract that from 220. That equals 178. Next, multiply 178 by 0.6 to get the low end of your training heart rate (106). Finally multiply 178 by 0.85 for the high-end rate (151). The formula is only an approximation. Anything between 106 and 151 would probably work well. If you don't like math, use the numbers in the accompanying chart to get in the ballpark. If you're just beginning, start at the lower range—or even lower if needed—and gradually increase the rate as you become more fit.

Aerobic Training Heart Rates

Brisk walking is enough to raise most people's heart rates into the aerobic range. At first, it won't take much effort at all to bump your pulse over 130. But as you grow more fit, you'll be able to do more without feeling winded. Don't overdo it. I encourage patients preparing for surgery to exercise, and I've had men come back to me and say "I walked two miles." "Great," I say, "and how long did it take?" "Well, an hour," they respond. Studies show that almost any exercise is better than nothing, but in this case, you've got to increase your speed to get the full cardiovascular benefits.

When you're working out at the right intensity for establishing aerobic fitness, you shouldn't be gasping for breath. You should be able to maintain a conversation and keep that level of intensity up for at least thirty minutes. But you should keep your pulse elevated for the entire time. The important thing is to establish a brisk pace and maintain it for an adequate length of time. Don't worry about distance.

PERCENT OF MAXIMUM HEART RATE						
AGE	60%	65%	70%	75%	80%	85%
25	117	127	137	146	156	165
30	114	124	133	143	152	161
35	111	120	130	139	148	157
40	108	117	126	135	144	153
45	105	114	122	131	140	149
50	102	111	119	128	136	144
55	99	107	116	124	132	140
60	96	104	112	120	128	136
65	93	101	109	116	124	132
70	90	98	105	113	120	127
75	87	94	102	109	116	123

Aerobic Activities	•	Walking
	•	Running
	•	Hiking
	•	Swimming
	•	Cross-country skiing
	•	Skating
	•	Dancing (Enjoy your partner and exercise at the same time.)
	•	Bicycling
	•	Machines (exercise bicycles, stair climbers, treadmills, rowing machines, ski machines, etc.)

Regular exercise works in concert with your balanced diet to boost your metabolism. So the amount of calories burned by exercise actually extends well beyond the time you spend exercising. Your body continues to burn more than its normal amount of fuel for hours after you finish a workout.

Ninety minutes a week is all it takes to enjoy most of the cardiovascular benefits of aerobic exercise, but a little more offers other benefits. If you start working out regularly and find you like it, try extending the sessions another ten minutes. Add a fourth day. Your fitness level will improve, and your body fat will start disappearing.

Regular exercise works in concert with your balanced diet to boost your metabolism. So the amount of calories burned by exercise actually extends well beyond the time you spend exercising. Your body continues to burn more than its normal amount of fuel for hours after you finish a workout.

Aerobic exercise of moderate intensity also has a unique ability to eliminate fat. During short sessions of exercise, your body depends on glycogen for energy, but after about twenty minutes of moderate exercise, it can access fat directly for energy to keep your muscles working. So the extra minutes beyond twenty minutes have special value. What's more, as you work out more and become more fit, you improve your ability to mobilize your fat stores increases. Dr. Neil Gordon, associate director of exercise physiology at the Cooper Institute for Aerobic Research, recommends that you walk three times per week for thirty to forty-five minutes in your target heart-rate zone to begin enjoying the full fitness and fat-fighting effects of exercise.

I enjoy a little variety in my aerobic routines. I run about four miles (thirty to forty minutes) a couple of times per week and spend about forty-five minutes on a stair-climbing machine or exercise bicycle over the weekend. The nice thing about using a machine is that I can catch up on my reading while I do it. On the other hand, I love running outdoors early in the morning. It's a great way to start a day.

This brings me to another great reason to work out longer. Exercise makes you feel good. Extended bouts of exercise release natural pain-relieving chemicals called endorphins in the body—what runners call "natural high." Endorphins might be one reason why people who exercise have a strong sense of well-being. But whatever the cause, psychologists recognize that aerobic exercise has many mental benefits. It relieves anxiety, decreases depression, lessens neuroses, and helps us cope with stress.

Strength Train to Build Hungry Muscles

Just as the image of tight female bodies in leotards leaping to and fro has given many people the impression that aerobic exercise is much more difficult than it actually is, bodybuilder competitions have given people a mistaken notion of what strength training entails. Most people think that weightlifting is for the Arnold Schwarzeneggers of the world.

In fact, not long ago, sports doctors did emphasize aerobic exercise over strength training for the average man—particularly the older man. But that attitude has changed dramatically in the last couple of years. The American College of Sports Medicine now recommends that all people strength train at least twice a week—along with sessions of aerobic exercise. And it's never too late to start.

Recent research has shown that older men can achieve muscular enhancement through weight training, in much the same way their sons, or even

Recent research has shown that older men can add muscle mass as rapidly as their sons.

grandsons, can. When a team of researchers led by William Evans, Ph.D., put ten ninety-year-olds from a nursing home on an eight-week strength training program, the researchers discovered that the men and women increased muscular strength, on average, by 174 percent. A report of their research in the *Journal of the American Medical Association* noted that the men actually enlarged their muscles significantly. They enjoyed healthier knees and increased walking speed 48 percent as well. More importantly, they were better able to get up and go about their lives.

For most of us, strength training is not a way to impress people at the beach, though looking good is a nice fringe benefit! It's a way to build muscles that help us stay lean—not to mention making life easier and more satisfying. Our goal here is to improve muscle tone, thus improving strength. You probably won't be entering many iron-pumping contests, but a properly designed weightlifting program helps you with everyday tasks such as hauling the groceries in from the car and yanking on the lawnmower cord.

> *Strong muscles protect your joints from injury and deterioration. And regular use of muscles dramatically slows the muscle atrophy that naturally occurs as we age.*

More importantly, strength training keeps your body in good working order as you grow older. Strong muscles protect your joints from injury and deterioration. And regular use of muscles dramatically slows the muscle atrophy that naturally occurs as we age. Strength training has also been shown to delay loss of bone density—osteoporosis—in older men. *In fact, exercise physiologists believe that some of the effects of aging can be postponed by as much as twenty years by strength training!*

The bottom line is that muscle helps keep you lean. Compared to muscle, fat is lazy tissue. It requires little energy to keep stored as excess baggage. So the more muscle you have, the more energy your body needs just to go about your daily routine. Fit people might use more energy than sedentary guys just sitting in a chair. That means they can eat more and still break even, and it means they've got significantly more energy for life!

Ten Tips to Strength Training

I strongly urge you to work with an experienced trainer at a gym to set up a program that suits your age, body, and activities. A session or two with an exercise physiologist can help you get much more from your workouts. They'll help you pick the optimal weight for you and show you how to do the exercises correctly, so as to help you avoid injuries. Ask friends for names of a good trainer. Use the same guidelines for selecting a trainer that you used when choosing a physician. *(Be aware of trainers who seem primarily interested in selling a club membership.)*

If you work out and *consistently* find yourself sore and hurting later, drop that exercise from your routine. Recently, I was having some trouble with my back, and I found that eliminating two sets of exercises helped ease the pain. Another good way to avoid injury, especially to the back, is to do what we call stomach crunches, which are modifications to the old-fashioned sit-up. They tighten the abdominal muscles, which are critical to building a flat stomach and preventing back injuries. Doing crunches is also a good exercise for a busy family to do together. We're shooting for forty or fifty a day. They take only a few minutes. There are ten basic rules to successful strength training:

1   Pick a weight that allows you to do eight to twelve repetitions before you're unable to lift it again.

2   Lift at least twice a week.

3   Settle on eight to ten exercises that work all the major muscle groups. (Upper body: chest, back, shoulders, abdomen, and triceps and biceps. Lower body: gluteus, quadriceps, hamstrings, and calves)

4   Focus on isolating the specific muscle groups. Many accidents happen when you use your back to jerk a

weight into position. Jerking usually means that the weight you're using is too heavy for the muscle group being exercised.

5 Do multiple sets after rest periods to increase the intensity; don't just add repetitions or weight.

6 Raise and lower the weight under control; never yank it up or let it drop. The motion you use while bringing the weight down is at least as important for building strength as the motion you use to lift the weight up.

7 If you like weight training, try split routines. Alternate your upper body and lower body muscle groups, or alternate large and small muscle groups.

8 Minimize rest periods between exercises so you will get some aerobic benefit from weight training. For example, you could alternate lower and upper abdominal crunches between sets.

9 Stretch muscles after each set.

10 Finish each session with a ten to fifteen minute aerobic workout (walking, running, cycling, stairmaster, rowing machine, etc.).

For most beginners, Nautilus-type machines work better because the machine eliminates any sideways motion that could cause imbalance and, therefore, perhaps injure you. But free weights can work just as well. Personally, I like both. I work out on machines at my health club a couple of times during the week, and I usually do a session of free-weight training with my sons at home over the weekend. Whichever approach you choose, never let the weight go all the way to the bottom, and never reach a point where your elbows or knees lock at the top. You want to keep pressure on the muscle at all times, not on the joint.

Finally, don't strength train more than three times per week, and take at least a day off between sessions. Building muscle is actually a process of damage and repair in the body, and you need to

> *Building muscle is actually a process of damage and repair in the body, and you need to give your body rest to allow it to rebuild and add muscle.*

give your body rest to allow it to rebuild and add muscle.

A New Way to Measure Success

For the first few months of your eating-and-exercise program, do me a favor and stay off the scale. First of all, if you did weigh yourself, you wouldn't see much change for several weeks, which could be discouraging. (Instant weight loss generally just shows that you're dehydrated.) But more importantly, pounds aren't the point. Being lean is. Muscles weigh more than fat, so if you're really successful, you might even gain pounds.

> *Pounds aren't the point. Being lean is. Muscles weigh more than fat, so if you're really successful, you might even gain pounds.*

The most accurate measure of fitness success is low body fat. You could have a trainer measure yours with skinfold calipers or a hydrostatic weighing. But a few percentage points one way or the other really don't matter. Most of us have ready access to the ultimate authority—a mirror and our own eyes. Take my word for it. You'll like what you see.

BODY FAT PERCENTAGE GUIDELINES (Howley and Franks Health Fitness, 1986)		
	Male	**Female**
Athletic individual	6-13%	14-20%
Fit	14-17%	21-24%
Overfat	18%	25%

(NOTE: Each percentage figure represents the amount of total body weight that is pure fat. You are allowed to carry more fat as you get older.)

 Q&A MAN TO MAN

QUESTION

How do you maintain a healthful diet when you travel and have to eat meals in restaurants with business associates?

ANSWER

I have a couple of simple tricks to keep my nutrition program in line when I travel. First, when I book my airline reservations, I always ask for low-cholesterol or vegetarian meals—not because I'm a vegetarian, but because I prefer the food. Again, sauces on the side only. Often, I'll get a nice, fresh fruit plate. Once I've reached my destination, I try to steer meals toward Japanese, Chinese, and southeast Asian restaurants, where the cuisine is generally pretty lean if you can avoid the sauces and fried foods. Remember, I always ask for my sauce on the side. Often, none is needed for a tasty meal. But if my taste buds demand some, I can at least control the quantity. These days, too, you can get grilled, broiled, or baked fish or chicken almost anywhere. Just be sure there's no sauce on top.

QUESTION	ANSWER

Much of what I read lately stresses how much more healthful a vegetarian diet is. Is that the ultimate goal?

I don't think you have to eliminate meat to eat well. In fact, it would be pretty boring for me. Also, the leaner meats—chicken, turkey, fish, and veal—are concentrated sources of protein. You can get that protein from plant sources, but you'd have to plan carefully and eat plenty. As long as you stick to lean meats and don't overdo it, I think a completely vegetarian diet is unnecessary.

There's an important distinction here, though. The nutrition plan I'm discussing will help prevent you from having health problems. But for people who already have problems—heart disease, for example—more extreme measures might be called for. Dr. Dean Ornish has had documented success reversing heart disease by cutting fat intake to around 10 percent of calories. To do that, he completely eliminated meat from his patients' diets.

Fortunately, you can still keep fat very low if you limit your daily intake of meat to no more than six ounces and select *lean* choices.

QUESTION	ANSWER

How do you deal with a sweet tooth?

I think I know this problem pretty well. Sweets do taste good, especially if you're used to eating them. But the boost you get from eating sweets is what makes them really attractive. When we sag in the afternoon, we look for a soft drink or a candy bar for a burst of energy. Deep inside, we know it's the wrong thing to do, but it does work—for a while. Sure enough, after an hour or so, we're dragging again, the sugar boost long gone. If you eat complex carbohydrates and eat them often enough—at least once every three hours—you won't feel the need for that sugar boost. And after you've gotten along without it for a while, you'll find that what used to seem pleasingly sweet now seems too sweet. Your sweet "tooth" is going away.

QUESTION	ANSWER
I like to work out at the gym on machines, but that's inconvenient when I'm on vacation or traveling on business. Is a week or so off that serious?	Exercise physiologists say that we begin to lose ground within about four days of stopping exercise, but a week probably isn't a serious infraction—as long as you really do start up again. That's the problem. Exercise is a habit, and you need to keep doing it to maintain the habit. Personally, I consider it the third most important thing in my life, after my family and my patients.

You really don't have to give up your workouts when you're away from the fitness center, though. Many hotels now have workout rooms or they have arrangements with a nearby facility. Ask when you make reservations. Every day, you can help keep yourself fit by getting exercise as you go about your business. Instead of riding elevators, climb stairs. Same goes for escalators. If it's going to take just about the same amount of time to walk or drive somewhere, why not enjoy the day? Exercise isn't only at the gym.

Ask your hotel staff for information on local walking/running trails and health clubs. Many hotels have maps of local trails. If you can't find a running trail, try some brisk walking at a local shopping mall. And going to and fro on your trips, try taking walks around the terminal while waiting between flights.

QUESTION	ANSWER
Which is better for strength training, machines or free weights?	*I like both.* I use machines at the fitness center I belong to, but I have freeweights at home. Dollar for dollar, you can do more with free weights than with machines. They're a good way for my wife, sons, and me to work out together. My expert friends tell me that machines are easier for beginners to use because they're easier to control and are generally *safer* if used properly. You also can't drop them on your feet. Free weights, however, aren't limited to a given repertoire of motions. Essentially, you can do anything with them that you can imagine.

HOTLINES	
American Dietetic Association	· **(800) 366-1655**
American Running and Fitness Association	· **(800) 776-2732**
Food and Nutrition Information Center	· **(301) 504-5719**
National Institute of Health (Nutrition)	· **(301) 496-9281**
President's Council on Physical Fitness and Sports	· **(202) 272-3430**

5

JUST SAY "NO"

**Warding off the
Ten Leading
Causes of Death**

MEN TALK : Mike Collins, age fifty

I can remember when it was considered strange for a man to take care of his body. Back in the fifties, when I was in high school, there were athletes and the rest of men. Of course, the athletes weren't necessarily the paragon of health. Muscles and a basic level of fitness were part of the 'jock' image, but so was a lot of drinking, drunk driving, and wild sex.

"So I suppose I was a bit of an oddball. I went out for track in high school—I've been running ever since—but I didn't get involved in most of the risky behaviors other guys did. My body has always been a part of me—not a tool separate from my brain—and I've tried to take the best care of it that I could.

"I've always been interested in my health, and have read what I could find that would help me preserve it. During the fifties it was odd to do that, during the sixties and seventies it was the exact opposite of what many men were doing, but by the eighties, the tide had begun to turn.

"Popular wisdom usually follows science by six to eight years, so I began to find interesting material on nutrition at universities by the early eighties. I had to dig for it, but I was interested, so I did. As a result, I've had a great life that's been free of any serious illnesses.

"We're in the midst of a fitness-and-health era now. The tools and knowledge to take care of yourself have not only become widely available, they're finally re-

spected. It only makes sense. The benefits of prevention are tremendous, and they only grow as we learn more."

> *For too long we—and I mean medical professionals and patients alike—haven't put enough value on staying in good health. We take it for granted—until we get sick. Then we look for cures.*

I can't think of a man who better exemplifies a preventive life-style than Mike Collins. He's attuned to his body, he watches for warning signs, he eats carefully, and he works out regularly. Not only that, he's been doing it for most of his fifty years.

The result? Mike might be fifty chronologically, but physically he's no more than forty. He has no health problems, he's fit, and he has an incredible amount of energy. At least as telling, he looks forty. In effect, I think Mike is forty.

Because of his smart choices in life, Mike has never had to learn that saddest of lessons: You don't know what you've got 'til it's gone. He's worked to keep his health, so he's never had to look back with regret on his vanishing powers. For too long we—and I mean medical professionals and patients alike—haven't put enough value on staying in good health. We take it for granted—until we get sick. Then we look for cures.

That time is past. Out of economic necessity, our nation is quickly recognizing the dollar value of preserving health. I don't think there's any question that most health-insurance plans will soon include prevention as a centerpiece of their programs. We'll all save money by heading off problems before they become life-threatening, but thinking of prevention strictly in terms of dollars doesn't give it enough credit.

By taking care of yourself, you'll do much to erase the seven-year difference in life expectancy between you and the woman in your life. According to Dr. Louis Sullivan, former Secretary of Health and Human Services, about 900,000 of the 2.2 million deaths in the United States each year are preventable. Your diet and exercise habits affect your likelihood of succumbing to fully four of the ten leading causes of death in men, and nine of the first ten are within your control to avoid.

Ten Leading	1	Heart Disease
Causes of Male	2	Cancer
Death	3	Accidents
	4	Stroke
	5	Lung Disease
	6	Pneumonia, influenza
	7	HIV Infection
	8	Suicide
	9	Diabetes
	10	Homicide

One study has found that 25 percent of men who were examined and found to have a potency problem related to poor blood circulation had a heart attack or stroke within five years.

We want a full, vigorous life, not some half-life stuck in a wheelchair or lugging around a colostomy bag. And that's the core of my message: Taking care of yourself improves the quality of your life right now. This is not just preaching or cheerleading; its based on hard scientific facts. That's why I told you about Dr. Lester Breslow's study in the last step. Dr. Breslow found that those who adopted what he called good health practices had considerably lower levels of mortality and disability than those who made health a low priority. Those who were living longer and better, Dr. Breslow learned:

- drank no more than two alcoholic drinks per day,
- didn't smoke cigarettes,
- kept their weight under control,
- slept seven to eight hours a night,
- were physically active,
- didn't eat between meals, and
- regularly ate breakfast.

Essentially, if you follow the recommendations in this book, you won't get old as soon. You'll have more energy—in the boardroom and the bedroom. Your brain does not exist in isolation from your body. If you want to be mentally sharp and full of energy, eat well and get fit.

And if you want to enjoy sex into your later years, that, too, requires that you maintain your body—which helps maintain your good attitude. The same sorts of bad health habits that give you heart disease—smoking, a fatty diet—can physiologically undermine your ability to get and sustain an erection. One study has found that 25 percent of men who were examined and found to have a potency problem related to poor blood circulation had a heart attack or stroke within five years.

It's not just physiological, though. The same bad health habits that tend to sap your erections also make you feel less energetic and less confident in yourself, which further erodes your performance. No one aspect—physiological or psychological— might be enough to make you impotent, but a combination of weights holding down your penis can easily do the job. Even if your efforts fall short and you do develop a health problem, it will be less severe. Your odds of recovering will be greater, you will suffer less, and you'll get better sooner. What's more, the very methods you used to reduce your risk will be instrumental in your recovery. I have observed that physically fit men who go in for surgery have fewer complications and get out of the hospital sooner. They can get back to their exercise routines sooner and their full recovery comes much sooner. Preventive strategies build on themselves to give you control over your health—control to stay healthier longer and get healthy sooner.

I constantly see men who have stopped acting as if good health just happens—and have decided to make it happen. Even if such men must undergo major surgery, they bounce back much faster than men who have let their health slide.

I constantly see men who have stopped acting as if good health just *happens*—and have decided to make it happen. Even if such men must undergo major surgery, they bounce back much faster than men who have let their health slide. So don't accept a decline in your health as fate. After all, "fate" and "fatal" come from the same Latin word. Accept your fate, and you could end up dead right. Why not, instead, take the simple, satisfying steps that will give you many more quality years?

Let me warn you about something: You're going to notice some repetition in this section. Why? Because many serious health problems stem from the same few causes. If you ignore basic maintenance of your car, eventually you get not just one, but all kinds of problems—brakes, engine, transmission, and more.

Similarly, too much booze, salt, or fat can hamper you in a number of ways. With that warning, and with your new health plans as a base, let's talk about how to avoid the leading killers of men.

The Terrible Ten

NUMBER 1

Heart Disease kills more than 350,000 men each year.

More than a third of all people who died in 1989 succumbed to heart disease. You can reduce your risk of following in their fatal steps by as much as 70 percent by doing the following:

Quit Smoking

One of the best bits of news for smokers is that your body can recover if you quit. When smokers give up the habit, their risk of heart attack drops 50 to 70 percent within five years.

I know what you're thinking—you want to quit, but how? I'm not making one absolute recommendation because there are a number of different ways to quit smoking—self-help groups, patches, Nicorete, hypnosis, etc.—and when there are multiple treatments being offered, that means there's no single cure that works for everyone. But somewhere out there is the cure that will work for you. Again, some of the same "investigative" tactics we discussed in Step Two for finding a physician will help you here.

Reduce your blood cholesterol level

Cholesterol in your blood is the villain that puts plaque on your artery walls, plugging them up so blood can't flow. Your body produces about two-thirds of the cholesterol that's in your blood, and the other third comes from the food you eat.

Total cholesterol—the combination of several different cholesterol-carrying components—has long been the most common way of talking about cholesterol. Unfortunately, we're learning that total cholesterol might be too simple an approach to heart disease. Although we know that men with total cholesterol over 240 are about twice as likely to die of heart disease as men with cholesterol lower than two hundred, reducing that risk might not be as simple as just lowering total cholesterol. Increasingly, evidence indicates that the ratio of the different components of the cholesterol equation are as important as or more important than the total. Refer back to Step Three if you're not familiar with HDL and LDL cholesterol; they appear to be a very important pair. The greatest risk reductions come from boosting HDL while you lower LDL, thus increasing the HDL:LDL ratio.

- You can improve your cholesterol profile by reducing dietary cholesterol and fat (especially saturated fat). A recent study suggests that an overall fat reduction and a switch to monounsaturated fats such as olive or canola oil is one of the most effective nonpharmaceutical ways to cut LDL (bad) cholesterol without cutting HDL (good) cholesterol at the same time. Pioneering work by Dr. Dean Ornish has shown that a very low-fat diet, combined with exercise and stress reduction, can even reverse the progress of heart disease. Recently, some insurance companies have recognized the importance of his program by agreeing to reimburse patients who enroll.

- Eating oat bran and fibrous foods (see Step Four for a list of high-fiber foods) also lowers cholesterol.

- Aerobic exercise is recognized as a good way to improve you HDL:LDL ratio.

- If those measures don't get your cholesterol into the healthful range, talk to your doctor about cholesterol-lowering drugs. Many people are having success using an inexpensive over-the-counter preparation of niacin, but you shouldn't take niacin without your doctor's advice. You need to be sure you take the right kind in the right amounts. Even if you do take niacin or other prescription cholesterol-lowering medications, watch your diet at the same time to maintain HDL.

- Maybe it should go without saying, but you can't reduce your heart-disease risk by lowering cholesterol if you don't *know* your cholesterol. Two-thirds of all people don't. Step Three describes cholesterol tests and what they mean.

Remember the man we talked about in Step One, who drove himself to the hospital during a heart attack? Afterwards he changed his eating habits and brought down his "bad" cholesterol from 250 to 190 through diet and exercise. He's now a happier, more confident man.

Keep your blood pressure within the healthful range.

For every point drop in diastolic (the smaller number) pressure, heart attack risk drops 2 to 3 percent. The American Heart Association now recommends diet and exercise as the first line of treatment for elevated blood pressure.

- Weight loss, and especially fat loss, have a direct effect on blood pressure. In one study, men who lost an average of sixteen pounds also lost an average of 4.2 points diastolic pressure. Exercise might produce even more dramatic results.

- Regular moderate aerobic exercise can cut diastolic pressure by ten points.

- People with blood-pressure problems also ought to go light on alcoholic beverages; one study of reformed Australian beer swillers saw an average drop in diastolic pressure of 3.3 points.

- Salt, too, is a culprit in some men. Perhaps as many as half of all men respond to excess salt with increased blood pressure. Talk to your doctor about the three-phase Salt Step Test, developed by the Blood Pressure Center in Washington, D.C.

- Be sure you eat plenty of fruits and vegetables rich in vitamin C. Studies have found that people with good vitamin C levels have average blood-pressure readings five points lower than those with the worst vitamin C levels (smokers).

Once again, you have to know you have elevated blood pressure before you can take corrective action. Don't be a part of the 59 percent who don't know those vital numbers.

I urge you to follow this advice, but as we were editing this step, a large study published in *The Journal of the American Medical Association* found that while diet and exercise were important in lowering blood pressure, the results were even better when medication was added.

Take one regular aspirin (325 milligrams or less) every other day, but not before you discuss it with your doctor.

Aspirin reduces the tendency of your blood to clot, cutting the risk of a heart attack by as much as 33 percent. But it also can cause other health problems, such as ulcers, and is not a good idea for people with bleeding disorders. Make sure you're okay before starting a regular aspirin program. I should mention that there is controversy as to the proper dosage, but don't think that if a little is good, more is better.

Eat foods high in vitamins C and E and in beta carotene. These vitamins are known as antioxidants, because they prevent unstable oxygen molecules from attacking living cells.

There is strong evidence that antioxidants—and especially vitamin E—help prevent LDL cholesterol in your blood from damaging artery walls and forming plaque. And they might even help clear plaque that's already in place.

VITAMIN C	VITAMIN E	BETA CAROTENE
Citrus fruit	Vegetable oils	Carrots
Tomatoes	Green, leafy vegetables	Green, leafy vegetables
Strawberries	Nuts	Broccoli
Green peppers	Whole grains	Squash

Because of studies that have been released in newspapers, many people are taking two to three times the RDA of these three vitamins (C, E, and beta carotene)

However, I should point out there are no long-term studies to date to show the benefits and risks of those higher doses. Certainly, this is a case where we can say that while a little is good, a lot might be bad. It is certainly possible to get too much of these vitamins. So be careful, don't go overboard, and ask your physician any questions you might have.

Eat a banana each day.

Potassium is emerging as a significant player in preventing hardening and thickening of arteries—particularly in people with blood pressure problems. One banana a day will give your vessels a protective friend.

NUMBER 2

Cancer kills more than 270,000 men each year

There is no question that heredity plays an important role in causing cancer, but many cancers also respond to what we call environmental effects. By that I don't mean just toxic chemicals; I mean everything we expose ourselves to. This includes natural and synthetic cancer-causing substances we eat, breathe, and touch; as well as various forms of radiant energy, from sunlight to radio waves to nuclear radiation. All of these influences

ESTIMATED NUMBER OF MEN DYING OF VARIOUS CANCERS IN 1993	
Lung	• 93,000
Prostate	• 35,000
Colorectal	• 28,800
Pancreas	• 12,000
Non-Hodgkin's Lymphoma	• 10,600

can start or encourage the growth of cancer. Fortunately, there are also substances that *inhibit* the start and growth of cancers.

The trick to successfully warding off cancer—and estimates are that most can be prevented (not cured, prevented!)—is to avoid things that promote cancer and emphasize those that inhibit it. The following strategies help you do both.

Stop using tobacco.   Smoking increases the likelihood of your getting lung cancer—the number-one cancer killer—by thirty-three times. But no matter how you get it into your body, tobacco dramatically raises your odds of getting cancer. Smoking tobacco causes lung and oral cancer, and has been associated with cancers of the pancreas, stomach, bladder, and esophagus; chewing it causes oral cancer; just being around people who smoke might cause as many as three thousand lung cancers per year in the United States. Quitting isn't easy—nicotine is more addictive than many people imagine—but it's the single most important thing you can do to protect your health. I try to get all my patients to stop smoking. But when I'm going to operate on a patient with cancer, I *insist* that he stop. There is no reason to risk a brush with death, recover, and then be stricken by lung cancer. It's like playing Russian Roulette, dodging the bullet, and then deciding to try it again.

No matter how long you've been smoking, your risk of lung cancer drops if you quit. Here's how a nonsmoker's and a quitter's risk of dying from lung cancer compares to that of someone who continues to smoke to age seventy-five and dies of lung cancer:

NONSMOKERS' RISKS OF DYING FROM LUNG CANCER VS. A 75-YEAR-OLD SMOKER	
Never smoked	• **33 times less likely**
Quit in thirties	• **10 times less likely**
Quit in forties	• **8 times less likely**
Quit in early fifties	• **5 times less likely**
Quit in early sixties	• **2 times less likely**

No matter how long you've been smoking, it's worth quitting and you can do it. Talk to your doctor, or the American Cancer Society, about the variety of programs to help people get off tobacco.

Test your home for radon gas, and correct the problem if there is one.

Radon is a naturally occurring radioactive gas that can enter your house from the soil. The Environmental Protection Agency believes that radon is second only to smoking in causing lung cancer. Simple tests can determine if radon is present in dangerous concentrations in your home, and modifications can be made to the structure to lower the concentration.

Consume no more than two alcoholic beverages per day.

Excessive alcohol consumption, besides causing cirrhosis of the liver, puts you at risk of colorectal, esophageal, and oral (especially if you drink beer) cancer. Although there is some evidence that light alcohol consumption is beneficial to your heart—it might increase HDL cholesterol—more definitely is not better. And remember, alcohol is the ultimate in empty calories. Aside from some B vitamins in certain beers, it has little nutrititional value.

Avoid unprotected exposure to sunlight.

Skin cancer is the most common of all tumors. More than six hundred thousand new cases of basal and squamous cell cancer and melanoma were reported in 1992, and the numbers are growing rapidly. Incidence of the most deadly form, melanoma, was up 80.6 percent and deaths increased 32.1 percent between 1973 and 1989. Sun exposure is the main cause of skin cancer, and there's no sign that its rampage is slowing. In fact, if ultraviolet radiation levels increase because of thinning of the earth's protective ozone layer, it's likely to accelerate. A Norwegian study has calculated that a 10-percent drop in ozone would increase melanoma by an additional 19 percent. At the Male Health Center, we've been involved in some cancer-screening programs with the employees of a large utility company—men who work mostly outside. Looking at the incidence of cancerous and pre-cancerous skin conditions among those men gives some scary evidence about what the sun can do. To help protect against skin cancer:

- Avoid direct sun exposure between 10:00 a.m. and 2:00 p.m.
- When you go outside for long periods, wear a sunscreen with a protection factor of at least fifteen, reapply it every two hours, and protect your skin additionally with a hat and clothing.
- Stay out of tanning parlors.
- Remember to do your self-exams. (Step One)

Go light on the fat. People who eat a lot of fat—most Americans—are more likely than their lean-eating counterparts to get several cancers. The connection appears strongest between colorectal cancer and fat, but prostatic, and perhaps even breast cancers, might also be more common in heavy fat consumers. (Yes, men can get breast cancer; I diagnosed one case the week I was working on this step.) Estimates vary, but it appears that low-fat fanciers may be as much as 50 percent less likely to get colorectal cancer, the number-three cancer killer of men. And a number of studies of Asian men who moved to the U.S. have shown that as they switch from the low-fat Oriental diet to a high-fat Western one, they get more prostate and colorectal cancers.

Take it easy on salt and salt-prepared foods. Besides boosting blood pressure in salt-sensitive people, salt has been linked to bladder and stomach cancer. Southeast Asian men, who enjoy a low rate of prostate cancer—perhaps because their diet is low in fat—are much more likely than American men to get bladder cancer, perhaps because of their penchant for salted and pickled foods.

Avoid unnecessary exposure to pesticides.

Research on the cancer-causing potential of pesticides is varied in its findings, because no one knows what the cumulative effects of exposure to routine pesticide use might be. However, some compounds that do seem to pose risks. Weed killers known as phenoxys (2, 4-D and 2, 4, 5-T, in particular) have been associated with problems in people who receive extensive exposure—such as chemical workers and farmers. They are more likely to develop a lymph cancer called non-Hodgkin's lymphoma. Weaker links have been made to cancers of the colon, lung, nose, and prostate. Also, recent research suggests a link between DDT and PCB, and breast cancer.

Beware of toxins in the workplace.

Back in the 1700s, men who cleaned chimneys for a living contracted a mysterious malady that was called "Chimney Sweepers' Disease"—scrotal skin cancer from the toxins that got inside their pants as they worked.

Today, we're starting to be more aware of cancer-causing dangers in the workplace. Although they don't account for a great percentage of cancers overall, you should know your risks on the job. Asbestos workers, of course, are notorious for their problems. But men who are exposed to cadmium on the job show increased incidence of prostate cancer, and vinyl chloride workers develop liver cancer at higher than normal rates.

Get lots of dietary fiber.

Fiber dilutes cancer-causing substances in your digestive tract and speeds them through, reducing the exposure. People who eat lots of vegetables and whole grains, which are rich in fiber, have lower rates of stomach and colorectal cancers. See Step Four for tips on getting your fiber.

Accentuate fruits and vegetables rich in antioxidant vitamins.

Antioxidants neutralize aggressive substances before they can damage genes and cause cancer. People who have high antioxidant levels in their blood are less likely to get lung, stomach, colorectal, esophageal, and oral cancers, but antioxidants might be important in preventing many other types of cancer. For example, researchers have found that people with low blood levels of vitamin A (of which the antioxidant beta carotene is one component) are more likely to get prostate cancer. Those with the lowest levels were at 2.2 times the risk as those with highest levels.

We're just beginning to understand the roles antioxidants play in our bodies. Other antioxidants, such as tannins, and substances that encourage them, might yet prove to be very important to cancer prevention. Just as exciting, we're starting to see applications of antioxidants in fighting existing cancers.

Exercise regularly.

Even strength training helps protect you, because it lowers the time food spends in your digestive tract.

A huge study of Harvard graduates has found that being active dramatically lowers your risk of getting colon cancer, and a study by Dr. Kenneth Cooper found a decrease in the incidence of cancer among fitter individuals. Even strength training helps protect you, because it lowers the time food spends in your digestive tract. So exercise protects you from colon cancer at the same time it keeps you from becoming constipated.

Take one aspirin every other day.

The same aspirin you take to lower your risk of heart disease (only after consulting your doctor) might also help prevent colorectal cancer. Some studies have shown that aspirin-like drugs inhibit the development of colon cancer from polyps (the precancerous growths) in animals, and people with arthritis, who take aspirin and aspirin-like drugs regularly, are less likely to develop colorectal cancer. That doesn't prove that aspirin prevents colorectal cancer. But you'll probably take it anyway, so you might as well enjoy the comfort of multiple benefits.

Know the warning signs and risk factors for various cancers.

The first step of this book gave you the tools to detect many cancers yourself and to know which ones you're most likely to get. Finding cancer early is vitally important. It increases your odds of survival, and it makes a cure much easier, less painful, and less costly. Testicular cancer, for example, used to be fatal much of the time. Now, though, with increased awareness of symptoms, more than 90 percent can be cured. The fatality rate dropped 63 percent between 1973 and 1989! There's no better proof that knowledge can save your life.

NUMBER 3

Accidents end the lives of almost 60,000 men each year.

Of the two sexes, there's never been any doubt which one is more accident-prone. White men can't jump, but they sure can wreck cars. Compared to white women, they're almost two and a half times as likely to die in a motor vehicle accident. It's the younger men, though, who really inflate the statistics. A man between fifteen and twenty-four is twice as likely to die in a car as men in general, boosting his risk to five times greater than the average woman. (Since my oldest son hit sixteen, I'm painfully aware of that every time I write a check for auto insurance.)

Of course, the car isn't the only place where men are at risk. Although automobile fatalities are dropping as cars have become safer, rates of accidental death of men from falls, drowning, fires, and firearms have remained steady over the last decade. In fact, if you combine deaths from firearm-inflicted accidents and homicides in Texas and Louisiana, you get a shocking statistic: In those two states, more people die from guns than die in motor vehicles—and needless to say, most of those getting shot are men. Furthermore, while more men know how to swim than women, five times as many men drown.

This is one area where tremendous improvements are possible, and progress starts between the ears. Whether you're climbing a ladder or swimming, don't assume you're too tough to be hurt, or that you can swim or fight or jump your way out of trouble. The world is full of sharp edges and deep water, and testosterone is not a bulletproof vest or a life preserver. I'm convinced that if we put away our bravado and our "It-won't-happen-to-me" attitude, men wouldn't suffer so many more accidents than women. Here are some ways we could start:

Don't drink and drive.

About half of all motor-vehicle deaths involve alcohol. Excessive booze is also involved in a high percentage of drowning deaths and boating accidents.

Wear a seatbelt— always.

There is no question that seatbelts save lives, and that goes for the back seat, too. A study in the *Journal of Trauma* has revealed that people in back seats die in accidents at almost the same rate as those in front. Why? Front-seat occupants are five times as likely to buckle up.

Consider getting airbags in your next new car.

Combined with lap and shoulder belts, airbags dramatically improve your odds of surviving a head-on collision.

If you ride a motorcycle or bicycle, wear a helmet!

You might believe in choice, but if you're smart, you'll choose to wear one. In California, motorcycle-related deaths dropped 38 percent in 1992, when they enacted a helmet law.

Be sure your home has smoke detectors and that they're working correctly.

Most people who die in house fires don't die from the flames; smoke suffocates them in their sleep. Smoke detectors can wake you up before it's too late.

If you have to have guns around, make sure everyone in your household knows how to handle them safely.

Trigger locks are one of the best ways to prevent firearm accidents. Keep your guns away from your kids!

NUMBER 4

Stroke took the lives of more than 56,000 men in 1991.

That's a grim figure in itself, but consider how many more are seriously crippled by stroke, the number-one cause of serious disability in the United States. More than 270,000 men suffer stroke each year, amounting to more than 1.2 million living men who've had strokes.

Stroke is a particularly debilitating disease. A heart attack can seriously cut into your physical capabilities, but stroke goes after your brain. When one of the arteries to your brain becomes plugged, you might be paralyzed on one side. Or you might lose sensation, memory, or the ability to speak or understand speech. Stroke victims often become completely dependent on others for survival. We're not often prepared for the ways that a stroke can announce itself. I saw a man in my office who complained of some weakness and numbness in his hand. The first episode lasted about an hour; the second, a week later, lasted about forty-five minutes. I sent him to a neurologist, who found he had a blocked carotid artery—the main artery that goes up the neck to the brain. An operation cleared the blockage, and might have saved him from a life-threatening stroke.

Fortunately, strokes can be prevented. Because more than 80 percent are caused by problems similar to those that cause heart attacks, many of the preventive steps you take to head off heart disease do double duty by also helping prevent stroke.

Keep your blood pressure within the healthful range.

Be sure you monitor your blood pressure regularly, and if it's elevated, follow the steps described in this section on heart disease to control it. Reducing your blood pressure to normal can cut stroke risk by 40 percent.

Avoid excessive alcohol intake.

Drinking more than a couple of alcoholic beverages per day raises your risk of stroke.

Follow all the steps for preventing heart disease.	People with heart disease are more than twice as likely to have a stroke.

- **Regular moderate exercise cuts risk 40 percent.**
- **An aspirin every other day reduces risk by 25 percent. (But don't take it without consulting your physician first.)**
- **Eating a banana each day cuts risk 40 percent.**
- **Getting plenty of beta carotene (an antioxidant vitamin) drops risk 40 percent.**
- **And one more time: stop smoking!**

Have a regular blood test for red-blood-cell count once you reach age fifty.	High levels of red blood cells thicken your blood, increasing stroke risk. The problem can be treated by taking blood thinners. (That's how aspirin helps prevent strokes.) In men, testosterone levels affect red blood cell count, and in fact, men treated for impotence with testosterone can have their blood count raised, although rarely to dangerous levels.
Have an electrocardiogram (EKG) every five years after age fifty to check your heart for atrial fibrillation, an irregular contraction of the heart.	This heart-rhythm problem is a serious risk factor for stroke and as many as one million Americans have it. Treating atrial fibrillation with medication reduces stroke risk by 80 percent. (See Step Three for a description of EKGs and what they mean. Also, refer to the chart at the end of Step Three for examination guidelines.)
Be sure your doctor listens to your neck with a stethoscope during checkups.	Blockage of the carotid arteries, the paired main arteries that go to the brain, plays a role in three-quarters of all strokes. If your carotids have heavy deposits of plaque, an operation can reduce stroke risk by almost two-thirds.
If you're African-American, start having tests sooner that warn of stroke risk.	African-American men are at almost twice the risk of dying from stroke as white men—probably because they are more likely to have high blood pressure.

Know the symptoms of mini-strokes.

Transient ischemic attacks (TIAs) are mild strokes that last from a few minutes up to twenty-four hours, after which the victim returns to normal. A person who has had one is at 9.5 times the risk of having a serious stroke later—one that can be prevented by getting prompt medical care. Symptoms include:

- temporary weakness, clumsiness, or loss of feeling in an arm, leg, or the side of the face on one side of the body

- temporary dimness or loss of vision, particularly in one eye

- temporary loss of speech, or difficulty in speaking or in understanding speech, particularly with right-side weakness

- sometimes dizziness, double vision, or staggering might occur

NUMBER 5

Lung disease cuts short the lives of almost 50,000 men each year.

Emphysema is included with chronic bronchitis under the catchall description *chronic obstructive lung disease*, but the fatalities are a result of emphysema. Emphysema is one of the simplest of all diseases to prevent—made all the more important because we don't know how to cure it.

Don't smoke; quit if you do.

Yes, I'm rubbing it in, but that's because smoking is the all-purpose bad guy. Most cases of emphysema are caused by tobacco smoke. It's a slow, lingering, and expensive way to die, usually bringing months and even years of impairment before death.

Avoid areas with heavily polluted air.

In this day of improving air quality, air pollution is unlikely to bring on emphysema. But those who already have lung problems ought to stay out of polluted areas if possible and certainly should avoid heavy exertion when the air quality is poor.

Wear a protective mask when you're in a dusty environment or are exposed to fumes.	Dust, sawdust, and other particles—as well as fumes—at home or in the workplace can irritate your lungs, bringing on emphysema or emphysema-like diseases.

NUMBER 6	**Pneumonia and influenza kill about 36,000 men each year.**

That is likely to be an unpleasant but temporary illness for a young man can be life-threatening to his father. As we grow older, we simply can't shrug off these infections with such ease. For that reason, older men need to take special steps to avoid becoming sick.

Everyone over the age of sixty-five should be vaccinated against influenza virus and pneumococcus bacteria.	Flu viruses usually start their annual march in late fall; see your doctor for vaccination against the season's prevailing types in late October or November if you're over sixty-five, or are at risk because of heart or lung disease, asthma, diabetes or immune disorders. Pneumonia vaccine is recommended for the same group of people at risk every six years.
Avoid exposure to people who have the flu or pneumonia.	Although it's not always easy, staying away from these bugs in the first place is the best form of prevention.
Keep yourself in good health by eating well and getting regular exercise.	A healthful diet and exercise boost your immune system, helping your body to fend off life-threatening illnesses and recover from them more quickly and easily. In one study at Johns Hopkins University, people who took a multivitamin got sick less than half as often as those who took no supplement.

NUMBER 7

More than 24,000 men take their own lives each year.

Despite the fact that they're twice as likely to suffer from depression, women commit suicide at about one-quarter the rate of men. Not only that, but there's some thought that many male suicides are actually misclassified as accidents because men are so inclined to take risks that threaten their lives.

Why are so many men dying at their own hands? Dr. Steve Manley, the psychologist who works with me at the Male Health Center, says that men are likely to blame themselves for problems. Instead of seeing depression and other psychological distresses as medical problems and seeking help, men are more inclined to believe their troubles result from their own weakness, lack of willpower, or some moral defect. Impotence is a prime example of a treatable physiological problem that can make a man depressed. Combine male pride with a serious lack of support systems for depressed men, and you have a lot of men who assume that nothing can be done. So they take matters into their own hands.

Dr. Manley says that some serious consequences flow from our insistence that men and boys be tough, stifle their emotions, and "play with pain"— not just on the football field in junior high, but in later life as well. Surprisingly, the era of the so-called Sensitive Man has done little to free men from these confining roles. The popular magazines and the talk shows proclaim that men are beating their drums and getting in touch with the hairy warrior inside them, but Dr. Manley sees few such "liberated" men.

Thankfully, Dr. Manley assures me that depression and other psychological problems that can lead to the extreme of suicide are readily treatable. They are medical problems that can be solved—if men speak up and seek help when they're unhappy.

Combine male pride with a serious lack of support systems for depressed men, and you have a lot of men who assume that nothing can be done. So they take matters into their own hands.

Often, progress can be made simply by getting men to ask themselves why they're feeling down. After all, life is more than a big "Smile" bumper sticker. We do run into problems and disappointments that bring us down, and we shouldn't expect to avoid them always. If you come home to find your wife in bed with a guy you thought was a friend, of course you're angry and sad. That's the right response to a bad situation. But if more minor things get you down, or the sadness lingers for weeks, do yourself a favor and find a doctor you can talk to.

Know the symptoms of major depression —for you and your loved ones.

Depression is marked by a loss of interest or pleasure in most normal activities, and one or more of several symptoms:

- **poor appetite**
- **disturbed sleep**
- **lack of energy**
- **loss of interest in sex and other pleasurable activities**
- **feelings of worthlessness and futility**
- **suicidal thoughts**

If you're depressed for an extended period, see your doctor and ask about medication.

In many cases, your general practitioner could help you emerge from your blues, either through discussion or by prescribing a mild antidepressant drug. Over half of all people who take antidepressants recover from their depression, although medication is not appropriate in cases where it's important to get at causes. Unfortunately, some doctors aren't well tuned to recognizing depression's symptoms—estimates are that half of depressed males go undiagnosed—so you might have to tell your doctor how you feel in order to get help.

Counseling can get you on the right track. There is no shame in therapy.

Problems are nothing to be ashamed of. Dr. Manley says more than half of depressed people can be helped within six weeks, either with psychotherapy—which is really just talking—or medically.

Get regular, moderate exercise.

What does exercise have to do with suicide? More than you might suppose. Moderate aerobic workouts are now recognized by psychologists as effective in fighting anxiety, stress, neuroses, and depression. In fact, it's even being recommended as a secondary therapy for severe depression.

NUMBER 8

As many as 14 million people worldwide might be infected with HIV, and more than three-quarters of them are men.

Until a cure is found, almost all people who catch human immunodeficiency virus will get acquired immune deficiency syndrome and die. So for the foreseeable future, prevention is the *only* way to save yourself from AIDS. There are three main ways to get it and three main ways not to get it.

Safe sex is not optional.

This issue is so important, I've made it Step Seven of this book. Please read it, believe it, and tell your son about it.

If you're facing surgery that might require a transfusion, consider banking your own blood in advance.

You must start four to five weeks before surgery, so your system has a chance to recover from giving blood, but the hospital can store three or four pints of your blood for backup. Ask your doctor about this procedure.

Don't use intravenous drugs and never, ever share a needle.

Shared hypodermic needles are the second-leading way that HIV is passed from one to another. It's not that I think that many drug users will read this book. But the fathers and mothers of potential drug users may, and your sons and daughters need to know the facts.

NUMBER 9

More than 20,000 diabetic men die each year.

Perhaps more than with any other disease, medicine has leaped forward during the past decade in its understanding of diabetes—the body's inability to properly process sugar. Diet, once considered only a way to control diabetes in people who already had it, has recently been recognized as a way to prevent or maybe even reverse many cases of diabetes.

Diabetes comes in two varieties, Types I and II. The first usually occurs during youth and requires insulin throughout life. The second, which is the variety I'll talk about here, usually occurs later in life and might come on very gradually. Experts estimate that only half the people who have Type II diabetes even know it. Nonetheless, their bodies are deteriorating. They risk blindness, heart attack, kidney failure, loss of a limb, impotence, and even death.

Know the symptoms of diabetes.

They come on gradually and they're easy to miss. Talk to your doctor if you've had two or more of these symptoms lately:

- **regular or constant thirst**
- **frequent need to urinate**
- **fatigue**
- **unexplained weight loss**

Get tested if you have a family history or symptoms of diabetes.

If you have a family history of diabetes, are more than twenty pounds over your recommended weight, or have high blood pressure or high cholesterol, you need to be tested. A number of different tests are available.

Keep your weight within the recommended range.

Obesity appears to be the most significant preventable cause of Type II diabetes. To get your weight under control, follow the instructions in Step Four.

Get regular aerobic exercise.

There it is again—the call of the gym. Exercise once again plays a significant and independent role in good health. In addition to its contribution to weight loss, moderate exercise improves glucose tolerance. In a study of twenty-two thousand male doctors, those who exercised at least five times a week were 42 percent less likely to develop diabetes than those who didn't exercise at all. And by combining a low-fat diet for weight loss and exercise, one study found that half of those men with early symptoms of diabetes were able to regain normal sugar metabolism and remain diabetes-free for five years.

Eat regularly.

Skipping meals is an invitation to blood-sugar highs and lows. Eat often—every three hours, ideally—to help keep your blood-sugar levels steady. You'll have more energy, and it will help your sugar processing system cope.

Reduce saturated fats.

It might be simply that saturated fat is the number-one contributor to obesity—the number-one precipitator of diabetes—but many studies show that reducing saturated fat helps control diabetes.

Eat foods rich in chromium.

Chromium is instrumental in the body's ability to regulate blood-sugar levels. Although studies conflict on whether supplemental chromium can prevent or reduce the severity of diabetes, evidence is strong enough for me to encourage you at least to eat foods that will supply the recommended dietary allowance of fifty to two hundred micrograms. Also bear in mind that people who exercise heavily may need more. You'll find lots of chromium in brewer's yeast, mushrooms, wheat germ, broccoli, and black pepper.

NUMBER 10

Homicide snuffed out more than 20,000 men in 1991.

For obvious reasons, we can't discuss homicide the way we have the other leading causes of death. The first nine of the Terrible Ten are within your control; you can do something to ward off all of them. Homicide, though, is something done to you, usually on a moment's impulse. There's no doubt, however, that some of the bulletproof macho attitudes we've talked about can play a major role in making some men killers and getting other men killed. Combine anger, alcohol, and guns, and you've got homicide waiting to happen. I don't have a magic wand, but I can say with confidence that men who follow the ideas in this book will find themselves happier, healthier, and safer.

One More Time, Now

To sum up, we've got to repeat ourselves. Smoking, diet, alcohol consumption, and other bad habits are the culprits here. They cause death and disability. But you can take your longevity and quality of life into your own hands by doing the things we've just talked about in this step. Also, get around to knowing your family history, doing your self-exams, and forming that health partnership with your doctor. You can do it. And it can make a difference. I've seen it happen.

 Q A MAN TO MAN

QUESTION	ANSWER
There's an awful lot to know when it comes to preventing disease. If you had to name the three most important things to remember, what would they be?	Two are easy, but the third—and it might be the most important—I'm going to hedge on a little bit. First, replace a large part of the saturated fat in your diet with complex carbohydrate. Second, establish a regular program of moderate exercise. And third, know the symptoms of life-threatening diseases and pay attention to your body for signs of them.

QUESTION	ANSWER
What about the "alternative" approaches to preventing or reversing heart disease, such as chelation, garlic, or a vegetarian diet? You haven't stressed these. Does that mean you don't think they work?	As for the first two you mention, I simply haven't seen enough research to endorse them. If I haven't got sound evidence to support a theory, I can't recommend it. On the vegetarian diet, however, we're starting to see some intriguing findings from Dr. Dean Ornish, whose work I mentioned earlier.

QUESTION	ANSWER
I tried using nicotine patches prescribed by my doctor to quit smoking, but I still ended up smoking again. Is it just impossible for some people to quit?	Statistics show that the longer you've been smoking, the harder it is to quit. But they also show that people in every category have succeeded. You didn't mention anything other than the patches prescribed by your doctor. Those patches are intended to be used along with a behavioral program that helps you quit. (Not psychotherapy, just some assistance in fighting the urge to smoke.) Without the support of a behavioral program, nicotine-patch users are much less likely to succeed in quitting.

QUESTION	ANSWER
The good news about aspirin is that it lowers your risk of colon cancer. The bad news is that it causes ulcers. What's a guy to do? Is there a happy medium?	Actually, there is. Aspirin appears to have a number of beneficial effects, including thinning the blood and possibly reducing the risk of colon cancer. An aspirin every other day is not likely to cause a problem with ulcers, nor is it likely to cause abnormal bleeding. (By the way, you should stop taking aspirin at least a week prior to surgery.) Certainly, if you are at risk for colon cancer or heart disease, an aspirin every other day is a reasonable consideration. However, it should be only a part of your strategy to reduce the risk of cancer or heart disease; exercise and nutrition should be an inte-

gral part of your strategy as well. Don't forget: Always check with your physician about the recommended dosage of aspirin.

QUESTION	ANSWER
Reading about depression always confuses me. Isn't everybody depressed from time to time? What's the difference between normal sadness and the kind of depression that you should get treatment for?	Of course we're all depressed from time to time, and that's perfectly normal. Without the valleys, we wouldn't appreciate the peaks so much. But when depression hangs on and begins to affect your functioning in your day-to-day life, or when you suddenly lose interest in things that have always given you pleasure, that's a different problem.

QUESTION	ANSWER
Eating smart and exercise and prevention are great, but everybody seems to have some uncle or grandfather who smoked two packs of Camels a day, drank a pint of bourbon every night, ate almost nothing but thick steaks and gravy—and lived to be ninety-seven. Isn't it really just luck or heredity? Why worry about it?	I hear those stories, too, and I'm certain that genes and luck play a big part in longevity—but how do you know you're the lucky uncle? Why gamble with the only life you've got? A very few people win the lottery. They quit work and live in luxury. But would it make sense for you to quit your job and wait for the big strike, just because you know *somebody* will win? What if it isn't you?

QUESTION	ANSWER
All this talk about environmental hazards, toxins, and cancer-causing agents sort of spooks me. What is the real threat out there and is there any way for me to protect myself fully?	Pollution of all kinds kills more than two million people worldwide each year. By 2000, an estimated three hundred thousand workers will die from disease related to asbestos exposure. More than fifty thousand U.S. workers die each year from chronic diseases associated with past exposure to toxins. The Environmental Protection Agency reports that for each one-degree decrease in our protective ozone layer, there is a two-percent increase in incidents of skin cancer. So the threat is real, and while there is no way to protect yourself totally, if you are in an environment where there are potential toxins, ask, inquire, and read. Be concerned and be alert.

QUESTION	ANSWER
There's no doubt stress has become pervasive in our society, yet as each year goes by, I suppose we become more "desensitized" to it. I want to get back in touch with just how much stress my body is feeling. What do you suggest?	Take some time off—a week, weekend, even an afternoon. I can tell just how much stress my body is under by taking at least a week off each summer and going off to Colorado with my family. I find it takes at least three or four days for me to start to slow down, and by the end of the week there is an incredible difference in the way I feel, my sleeping habits, and my relationship with my family. I find that even a long weekend can do me a lot of good.

HOTLINES	
American Cancer Society	· **(800) 227-2345**
American Council on Alcoholism	· **(800) 527-5344**
American Diabetes Association	· **(800) 232-3472**
American Heart Association	· **(214) 706-1179**
Cancer Information Service (NIH)	· **(800) 422-6237**
Environmental Protection Agency	· **(800) 621-8431**
National Council on Alcoholism and Drug Dependency	· **(800) 622-2255**
National Injury Information	· **(301) 504-0424**
National Institute of Mental Health	· **(301) 443-4513**
National Pesticide Telecommunication	· **(800) 858-7378**
Office on Smoking and Health	· **(404) 488-5701**
Radon Hotline	· **(800) 767-7236**
Suicide Crisis Line	· **(800) 621-4000**
U.S. Consumer Product Safety	· **(800) 638-2772**
U.S. Government Occupational Safety and Health Administration	· **(800) 356-4674**

6

KEEP IT UP

**Maintaining
Sexual Intimacy
Throughout a
Longer Life**

MEN TALK: Cliff Davison, age sixty-five

L ooking back, I guess I'm just about a perfect example of how to get impotent. I ate badly and I
was too busy at work to get any exercise. Well, it
caught up with me in a big way. When I was about
sixty, everything seemed to start falling apart.

"First, I had a prostate problem that required an
operation, and nine months after that, I had a heart
attack. At the same time—even before—you see, I was
having some problems in the bedroom. I was interested in sex, and I could get an erection. But it wouldn't
stay around long enough to satisfy my wife.

"After a couple of failures, I started avoiding sex.
I'd go to bed early or late, and I'd try not to touch her.
We didn't talk about it. It was like part of our life
together just shut down.

"I brought it up to my regular doctor one time during a
physical, but he just said, 'You're getting older; that's just
what happens.' At the time, I guess there was something
that didn't ring right about that, but I didn't know how
wrong he was until I went back for a check-up to the urologist who did my prostate surgery. He wondered how things
were going, and then he flat out asked, 'Any trouble in the
bedroom?' (I guess he knew a guy in my situation was
likely to be having erection problems.)

"I admitted that I just couldn't keep it up, expecting
a pat on the back and condolences. Instead, he said,
'We've got lots of different things to try. There's no rea-

son for you to live with the problem.'

"I tried some yohimbine pills and erection injections. The pills might have helped a little, but they weren't enough. Injections really did the job, but I just couldn't get comfortable with the needle.

"For me—for us, I should say—the vacuum device is great. It's simple, painless, and it works. I need to plan ahead a little, and it does require a pause in sex if I don't put it on in advance, but that's turned out to be no big deal. I guess I was sort of surprised, but my wife doesn't mind at all. Since I got some help, we've started talking a lot more. I came to find out after all these years that she doesn't really have inhibitions about what we do behind closed doors. She's been very supportive. She says the fact that I feel better makes her feel better. And you know, I think when she feels better, I feel even better. It sort of builds, and it's got as much to do with the talking as the sex.

"As a matter of fact, I'm talking to all sorts of people about it. I started going to this support group of guys with erection problems. I expected it would be a bunch of old duffers, but there were men in their thirties and forties there—all talking about what had happened to them. Then recently, I was playing golf with a very good friend. He sort of skirted around telling me, but I figured it out. When I told him I had the problem, too, he said, 'It's good to hear that. I was beginning to think I was the only one in the world.'

"Getting this out in the open and getting help has made an amazing difference in my life overall. I'm inspired to take care of myself now—I'm eating well and getting exercise—because I want to be around a while longer to enjoy life."

Living longer is a fine goal, but you might have noticed that the title of this book includes the word "better." Isn't that our real goal—to live not just more years, but *better* years? There's more to life than numbers of years, pounds of weight lost, miles run, or even dollars saved. While you're doing those things, you should be enjoying yourself. And one of the most fundamental pleasures we have is sex. It is one of God's gifts—an endowment we should take advantage of and enjoy fully.

Human sexuality is not just a hard penis and ejaculation. Sex sets us apart from other species because for us it is more than just reproduction. As Dr. Dudley Danoff says in his helpful book *Superpotency*, good sex has many benefits beyond just feeling good. These include:

- It's a natural tranquilizer.
- It's great physical exercise.
- It helps with cardiovascular fitness.
- It stimulates the nervous system and the prostate gland, and clears out mental cobwebs.

A patient once told me a grim joke about impotence: "Do you know the difference between worry and panic? Worry is the first time you can't do it the second time. Panic is the second time you can't do it the first time."

Sadly, a Boston University study says that at least thirty million American men are functionally unable to share the joy of intimacy because they are impotent. Impotence—the inability to attain or maintain an erection sufficient for the mutual satisfaction of both partners—is one of the most psychologically devastating problems a man can have. That's why I'm devoting this long step to its causes and cures. Much of this book is devoted to helping you live longer; but I want you to enjoy life to the fullest along the way.

A patient once told me a grim joke about impotence: "Do you know the difference between worry and panic? Worry is the first time you can't do it the second time. Panic is the second time you can't do it the first time."

We both laughed, but we all know that sexual failure is no joke. From our middle teen years onward, sexuality is probably our strongest preoccupation. That preoccupation can bring pleasure, closeness, and security, or it can bring frustration, isolation, and fear. I've seen good marriages torn apart by impotence. Impotent men and their partners—yes, she suffers equally—often lead miserable, incomplete lives.

At the Male Health Center, I see many men so shattered by impotence that they can't even make eye contact with me. Then, as they progress toward sexual health, a miraculous change comes over them. They talk differently; they even walk differently. As one of my patients recently told me, trouble in bed can affect almost every aspect of our lives. "The problem with impotence is not just that a piece of flesh doesn't get hard," he said. "The problem is how that failure affects that person and his relationships with the people around him, his children and his family."

He went on to say that his impotence even affected his job performance.

"With very little self-esteem, it's hard to be positive at work," the man said. He believed that in an effort to regain his lost sense of worth as a man, he became overly aggressive and "pushy" at work. "I was trying to make up for a sense of inadequacy, and I stepped on the wrong toes."

What a pity. And it's all so unnecessary.

It's easy to overlook the damaging effects of impotence on a man's partner. Too often, the man alone is seen as the patient and his partner is barely acknowledged, or merely tolerated. That's wrong, guys. A woman, raised on the same myths of men as highly sexual and always ready to perform, might see her partner's erection as an emotional lie detector—the only real proof that a man loves her or desires her. So no erection, no love. If he's not erect, she thinks, he must not find her attractive. We'll talk much more about this in Step Eight.

With the capabilities of modern medical science, any man can have an erection. Yes, even a quadriplegic man—paralyzed from the neck down and unable to feel anything in his penis—can have erections. So don't imagine that loss of erections is a normal part of aging. Don't think that you're alone

> *Too often, the man alone is seen as the patient and his partner is barely acknowledged, or merely tolerated.*

and nothing can be done. There is help—for every man who'll take it.

Simply restoring function, however, won't guarantee that you will have the best sex you can have. In fact, many men with fully functioning penises are not having the best sex. In the following pages, we'll talk at length about getting and keeping erections. But before we do, I think we better have some idea how we plan to use those erections to our best advantage.

The Sexual Arena

The message we get from the media ... If you aren't twenty-five, ten pounds underweight, with a bushy head of hair and a ten-inch, rock-hard penis that works like an automatic garage door, you can't have good sex.

Nothing is more important than sex to a man's self-esteem. Sadly, our society has defined and distorted sex until it's often a destroyer of self-esteem. Wherever a man turns these days, he's encouraged to think of sex as performance and to compare his performance to unachievable fantasies.

Where do we find the American model of sexuality? In men's magazines—where the women and men are all perfect. You don't even have to look at men's magazines; just look at your Sunday newspaper or any advertisement. These men and women are thinner, more athletic, and better looking than ninety-nine out of a hundred real people. The message we get from the media, like the message that we get from so many advertisements and from most of our show-biz personalities, is this: If you aren't twenty-five, ten pounds underweight, with a bushy head of hair and a ten-inch, rock-hard penis that works like an automatic garage door, you can't have good sex.

And how do we define good sex? It's conquest. Scoring. We've reduced sexual intimacy to chiseling notches in a pearl-handled revolver. We have a few winners—the glamorous superstuds with their perfect women—and lots of losers: the rest of us who drive ourselves crazy trying to live up to these false images. It is a male attitude, one of several we'll discuss in the conclusion, that dominates our culture. Is it any wonder that boys think they can become men by forming "posses?"

Great sex is within every man's reach, but it is not a given.

Stop a minute to think about it, though. Do our sexual idols really have better sex than we do? The evidence suggests not. On the contrary, they appear to divorce regularly, and abuse drugs and alcohol—and none of that is conducive to having great sex.

In fact, the keys to better sex now and in your later years are a strong relationship, a healthy body, and self-respect. And just as any of us can improve our relationships, our health, and our attitudes, so can any of us have better sex.

But let me not oversimplify. Great sex is within every man's reach, but it is not a given. As Bernie Zilbergeld, Ph.D., says in his landmark book, *The New Male Sexuality*, "Good sex is no more doing what comes naturally than is adult conversation. Virtually all of the men and women I've talked to over the years who say they have good relationships and good sex report that they had to unlearn or give up a number of harmful notions, and replace them with ideas that were more realistic and constructive."

What are those harmful ideas? Zilbergeld points out in his book a dozen destructive myths about sex (summarized in the conclusion of this book), but the notion of sex as performance is the one I want to concentrate on here. In my medical practice, I help men overcome problems with erections, premature ejaculation, and other sexual difficulties. And I've found that the single most destructive force is the belief that sex is some kind of competitive sport. When a man believes he must live up to some imagined and unrealistic standard of sexual excellence, he's going to feel considerable anxiety. And that anxiety can wreck his sex life.

When a man believes he must live up to some imagined and unrealistic standard of sexual excellence, he's going to feel considerable anxiety.

In the following pages, we're going to talk in great detail about physical causes for male sexual problems. Indeed, you'll learn that more than half of all potency problems have a treatable, physical cause. But every man who has had an erection problem also has an emotional problem. And that anxiety—

> *I'm convinced that many of my patients—although their ability to have erections might be physically compromised to some degree—could have successful sex if they could just feel relaxed and confident.*

that fear that he might fail again—sets him up for future failure. There's nothing mysterious about it. Fear produces chemicals in our bodies that stop erections—immediately!

For that reason, I never look at sexual problems as merely physical. I'm convinced that many of my patients—although their ability to have erections might be physically compromised to some degree— could have successful sex if they could just feel relaxed and confident. Drugs or surgery can't accomplish that. It requires treating the whole man.

Through sex, we show caring, we give, we receive pleasure, we share what might be the most fundamental fun, and, yes, we create new lives together. Those human, emotional qualities—not just physiological responses—make sex good.

The Penis—An Owner's Manual

Considering that about half of all people have one, I'm amazed at how few of the men I see actually know how a penis works. Too bad, because that knowledge has a lot to do with keeping one working correctly.

It's important to understand that there are two distinct aspects to male sexual response: erection and ejaculation. Although they happen in the same part of your body, they are very different processes. They are controlled by nerve centers in different parts of your spine, under direction of the brain, and one response can happen without the other. (Yes, to answer the question I'll bet you're asking, you can ejaculate without having an erection.)

What makes it go up?

You can think of the process of getting an erection as the equivalent of filling a tire with an air compressor. (Figure 1) The main difference is that the penis fills with blood rather than air. To get the job done, you need a good control switch (brain), well-insulated wires (nerves), a strong compressor (the heart), an adequate supply line (arteries), and a tire (the penis) without leaks (veins) .... If any of these components are defective, you've got a flat tire. (Figure 2)

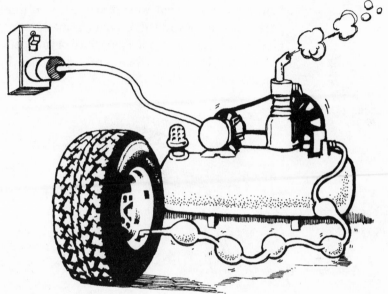

Figure 1

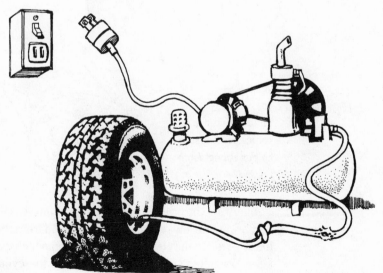

Figure 2

Underneath the skin on the penis, an elastic layer called the tunica albuginea encloses three cylinders—two on top that are connected and composed entirely of blood-vessel tissue, and one on the bottom, through which urine passes. All three of these cylinders, called corpora (cavities), extend inside the abdomen—about one-third of your penis is actually inside you—and are surrounded by muscles. (Figure 3)

Anatomy of a Penis: *Figure 3*

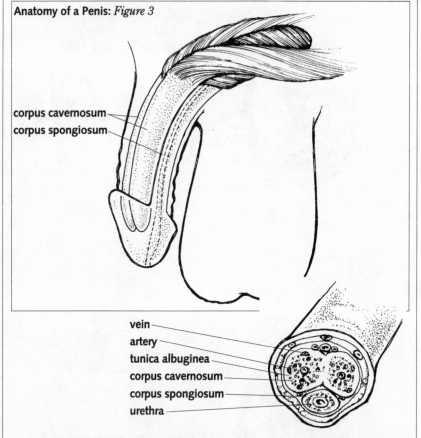

corpus cavernosum
corpus spongiosum

vein
artery
tunica albuginea
corpus cavernosum
corpus spongiosum
urethra

Arteries—the progressively smaller blood vessels that bring nutrient- and oxygen-rich blood from the heart—run up the center of each of the upper chambers. Branches supply storage areas in the cylinders called lacunae (lakes), and veins—the vessels that carry used blood back to the heart—exit the lakes, pass through the tunica, and run back inside the abdomen under the skin. (Figure 4)

Flaccid (Non-erect) Penis: *Figure 4*

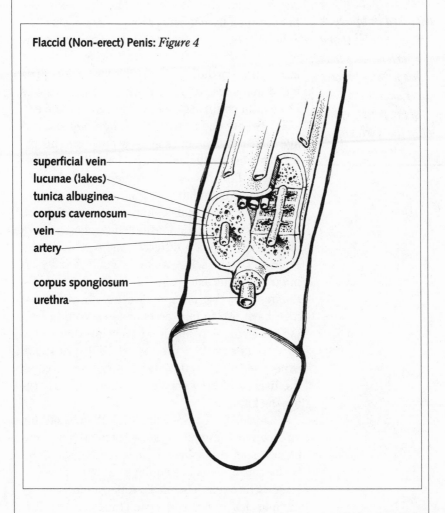

- superficial vein
- lucunae (lakes)
- tunica albuginea
- corpus cavernosum
- vein
- artery
- corpus spongiosum
- urethra

Most men have two to four erections every night lasting fifteen to thirty minutes each while they sleep, as we've discussed in previous steps. (At least one expert believes that this nightly process nourishes the tissues of the penis, somewhat like recharging the batteries.)

As you go about your normal daily activities—presumably without an erection—the arteries (the supply lines) are relatively small and very little blood enters the lakes (the inner tube). Why? Here's the tricky part. Blood flow remains minimal (just enough to keep tissues alive) because muscle tissue in the penis stays tense. I know it sounds odd, but having a flaccid penis requires tense muscles, although you aren't aware of them. Those muscles, which are within the walls of the arteries and lakes—prevent the lakes from filling with blood. The blood that does enter the penis to nourish tissues flows right on through without much resistance.

For twenty-one or twenty-two hours of an average man's day, the muscles stay tense and his penis stays neatly tucked away. Three things, however, can flip the switch. Some sexual thought might enter his mind, causing nerve impulses to travel down his spinal column. Or, there might be some direct stimulation to his penis, causing nerve impulses to travel a different pathway up to the brain and then back down to the spine. Finally, he might be sound asleep and his brain might trigger the impulses that bring on erection. In fact, most men have two to four erections every night lasting fifteen to thirty minutes each while they sleep, as we've discussed in previous steps. (At least one expert believes that this nightly process nourishes the tissues of the penis, somewhat like recharging the batteries.)

Whatever the cause, when the call goes out for an erection, a complex reaction begins. Nerve impulses from the spinal column, mediated by the brain, cause the nerve endings in the penis to release nitric oxide. The nitric oxide, in turn, causes the muscles in the arteries and the lakes to relax. The arteries expand, increasing flow, the lakes fill with blood, and an erection is on its way. (Figure 5) (A second set of nerves releases chemicals that cause those muscles to tense again, quickly wilting an erection. As you'll see shortly, when this switch gets flipped at the wrong time, you've got a problem.)

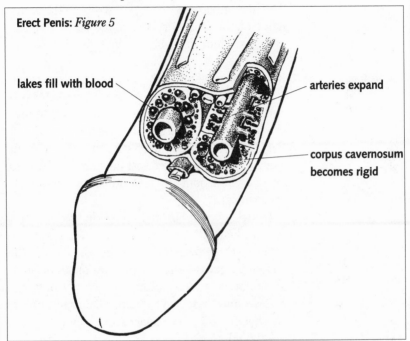

Erect Penis: *Figure 5*

lakes fill with blood

arteries expand

corpus cavernosum becomes rigid

As they expand, the lacunae compress the veins that normally carry blood out of the penis against the tunica, restricting flow out of the penis. The resistance to the flow of blood out of the penis increases dramatically. Pressures inside the penis exceed the peak pumping pressure of your heart, and when the muscles that surround the cavities contract near the peak of arousal, the pressures go even higher. Additionally, squeezing the head of the penis—primarily in the vagina—might further increase blood pressure.

In any event, as long as the switch stays on, the nitric oxide flows, the pressure stays high enough, and leaks don't develop, your tire will stay inflated. That's *how* erections work, but it's also worth considering *why*. Although they don't play a direct role in causing an erection, hormones secreted by the testicles and the adrenal gland do control our interest in sex and our level of arousal. The levels of these hormones are seldom steady, so our sex drive varies. To be honest, we don't know where these hormones work in the brain or in the penis, but they clearly are indispensable to a vibrant sex life.

Ejaculation

Most of the men I see, whether it be for vasectomy or impotence, believe that the testicles provide the fluid that makes up semen. In fact, though the testicles do produce all the sperm in semen, they contribute less than 5 percent of the volume overall. Still, since they're at the bottom of things, let's start our journey through the reproductive tract there.

Testicles begin life well up inside the abdomen and gradually descend as the fetus nears birth. In rare cases, the testicles fail to descend outside the abdominal cavity before birth. The condition needs to be corrected surgically because not only can undescended testicles fail to produce sperm properly, but the risk of testicular cancer is much greater.

Although more men worry about penis size than testicle size, it's not unusual for a man to be concerned that small testicles might mean he's less manly. As one who has seen and held countless thousands of them, let me assure you that testicles come in a wide variety of sizes, and bigger does not mean more virile. And while we're on the subject, it's perfectly normal for one testicle to be larger than the other, and one will usually hang lower in the scrotum. (By the way, men can still function well if they lose one testicle; it's like driving without a spare tire.)

The testicles have two main purposes. First, they produce between 60 and 65 percent of testosterone (the male sex hormone) and secrete it into the blood stream. (The remainder is produced in the adrenal gland.) Testosterone gives us our sex drive, makes erections possible, controls male characteristics such as facial hair, and serves numerous other purposes.

As one who has seen and held countless thousands of them, let me assure you that testicles come in a wide variety of sizes, and bigger does not mean more virile.

And, of course, the testicles produce sperm—the male contribution to future generations. Sperm start off as tiny tubular cells that take more than seventy days to be transformed into something close to the finished product.

But sperm, as they emerge from the testicles, aren't yet ready for prime time. They need to mature and grow stronger in the epididymis, an assemblage of tubes attached to the back of each testicle. (Figure 6) Completely uncoiled, the epididymis might measure twenty feet in length, yet it is little more than a half-inch wide, and two to three inches long in its compact version.

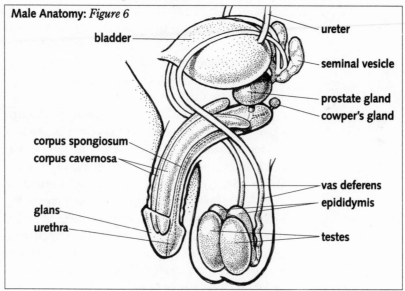

Male Anatomy: *Figure 6*

bladder — ureter — seminal vesicle — prostate gland — cowper's gland — corpus spongiosum — corpus cavernosa — vas deferens — epididymis — glans — urethra — testes

Once they reach the end of the epididymis, sperm are mature and able to swim actively by wiggling their tails. They then travel up the vas deferens, which are tubes about as thick as large spaghetti and roughly a foot long, with pin-hole passages through which sperm travel. The vas are the pipelines we cut and block off during vasectomy. The vas finds its way out of the scrotum along the spermatic cord, which includes the vas deferens and blood vessels.

Just short of the prostate gland, the vas deferens widen into the ampulla, a kind of launching pad where sperm wait for the opportunity to be ejaculated. The seminal vesicles lie behind the prostate and the bladder, and supply a fructose-rich (rich in sugar) mixture to the ejaculatory fluid to support the sperm on their reproductive journey. Combined with sperm from the testicles, prostatic fluid from prostatic ducts, and seminal fluid from the seminal vesicles in the urethra, this fluid makes up what is usually called semen.

Before the semen spurts from the urethra, however, the Cowper's gland secretes a small amount of watery fluid into the urethra. This is usually present at the tip of the penis during arousal and prior to ejaculation. Although we're not certain what purpose it might serve, it's likely the Cowper's gland secretions lubricate the inside of the urethra to make way for the semen.

Semen flows into the urethra shortly before ejaculation, which is accompanied by increasing muscle tension in the pelvic area—the feeling that ejaculation is imminent and irreversible. (We'll talk more about this when we discuss premature ejaculation later.) Signals from a nerve center in the spinal column go out to muscles in the pelvic area. The bladder neck closes, to prevent the semen from going into the bladder, and the muscles that surround the corpora inside the abdomen contract powerfully to expel the semen.

Shortly after ejaculation, the components of the semen react, changing in consistency and forming a protective medium for the sperm in the woman's vagina. If everything else goes as designed, fatherhood is the result.

How Big, How Hard, How Often?

Most men aren't as interested in how the penis works as they are in *whether* it does, how *often* it should, and how *big* it should

Because the vagina is quite versatile in accommodating various penis sizes, your length and circumference have nothing to do with satisfying a woman. The size and shape of a man's penis when not erect does not indicate how large it will be when it is erect. Differences disappear behind closed doors.

it be. I constantly see men who worry about measuring up to someone else's yardstick, whether in size or studly performance. As I've already pointed out, this is exactly the wrong attitude to carry around if you want to improve your sex life. It centers on hardware rather than emotions. But such concerns are not unusual, and the facts can help ease the worry.

First, because the vagina is quite versatile in accommodating various penis sizes, your length and circumference have nothing to do with satisfying a woman. You might not know that most penises, when erect, measure about six inches long—or, as Dr. Dudley Danoff's patients often put it, "half a foot." The size and shape of a man's penis when not erect does not indicate how large it will be when it is erect. Differences disappear behind closed doors.

Some of this misunderstanding stems from the fact that men tend to think of erections as "on" or "off"— either fully flaccid or hard as a telephone pole. Think about it, though, and you know that's not the case. For example, even when you're not aroused, your penis shrinks and expands in response to temperature changes. Likewise, erections are far from absolute—they are not like automatic garage doors. When we talk about their quality at the Male Health Center, we rate erections on a scale of one to ten—with one being flaccid, five being just sufficient for intercourse, and ten being what one of my patients calls "a diamond-cutter"— the single stiffest one you ever had (most likely when you were considerably younger than you are today).

Which brings us to a very important point: It is absolutely normal for your erections to change as you grow older. You don't expect to be able to run the mile as fast when you're fifty as you could when you were twenty, and you shouldn't expect your penis to respond as quickly either. That doesn't mean you'll enjoy sex any less at fifty. Quite the opposite: You can enjoy it more when your body gives

> *She needs to understand that when you don't become rock hard at the sight of her, that has nothing to do with how attractive you find her. It's just normal change.*

you time to relish the pleasure. You'll run that mile slower, but you might enjoy the scenery more.

As you grow older, your penis will not point upward as much when it's erect. You can also expect to require more stimulation to achieve an erection. At twenty, a fleeting thought might do the job, but as we age we're less likely to become erect in response to an erotic thought or image. Your partner needs to understand that more direct physical stimulation is needed. Likewise, she needs to understand that when you don't become rock hard at the sight of her, that has nothing to do with how attractive you find her. It's just normal change.

Couples also have sex less often as they grow older, which just reflects the fact that the hormones that control our sex drive decline somewhat as we age. But they *do not* go away! Many people continue to want and have sex throughout very long lives. In fact, Masters and Johnson have found that 30 percent of seventy-year-olds continue to have sex at least weekly (not weakly), and 60 to 70 percent have sex at least monthly. Having less sex is normal when we grow older, but having sex and enjoying it is absolutely normal. Impotence is not a fact of aging.

> *Masters and Johnson have found that 30 percent of seventy-year-olds continue to have sex at least weekly (not weakly), and 60 to 70 percent have sex at least monthly.*

Most sexual functions happen more slowly as we put on years, and that's not all bad. Although it might take you longer to get an erection, and you won't be able to get another one as quickly after ejaculation, you're also likely to take longer to ejaculate in the first place—extra time to share pleasure and intimacy. Combine that with fewer distractions from children around the house, and you might find that you spend nearly as much time having sex as you did when you were younger, although you do so less often.

You're probably wondering when these changes will take place. Will your erect penis drop to horizontal when you turn forty-eight? Will you have sex 1.73 times per week when you're sixty-four?

I could tell you what the averages are, but they

Dr. Irwin Goldstein, a Boston University urologist and world-renowned expert on impotence, believes that the oxygen-rich blood that fills your penis when it becomes erect helps keep the tissues in the organ healthy and flexible, maintaining their ability to stretch, fill with blood, and produce an erection. So in a very real way, your ability to have an erection is a "use it or lose it" proposition

wouldn't mean anything to you, because you're not average. By following the advice in this book, you're going to postpone these changes dramatically. People who take care of their bodies by eating well, exercising, and practicing preventive medical care can forestall physical decline by ten to twenty years. No, you can't stop your hair from falling out by cutting the fat in your diet and taking up running. But you can keep your body (and penis) working better. In effect, you can have at sixty the body and sex life of a man forty-five years old.

We've also learned recently that this healthful process tends to build on itself. When you stay fit and healthy, you have more erections and more sex. And getting erections preserves your ability to have erections. Dr. Irwin Goldstein, a Boston University urologist and world-renowned expert on impotence, believes that the oxygen-rich blood that fills your penis when it becomes erect helps keep the tissues in the organ healthy and flexible, maintaining their ability to stretch, fill with blood, and produce an erection. So in a very real way, your ability to have an erection is a "use it or lose it" proposition.

When The Tire Goes Flat

Taking care of yourself greatly reduces the likelihood that you'll have a sexual problem, but it still can happen. As many as thirty million men in America (at least one in four) are impotent—they're unable to get or keep an erection stiff enough to have intercourse. Significant curvature of the erect penis—called Peyronie's disease—is much less well known, yet might be more common than what we had thought. Another devastating difficulty—premature ejaculation—thwarts the sex lives of about thirty-six million men, studies show, yet few men who are affected seek help to overcome it.

Thirty million . . . thirty-six million . . . we better cherish what works, guys.

Thankfully, all of these conditions are treatable.

In fact, each has a number of solutions. If one of them is bothering you, read the following paragraphs—*but don't stop there! See your doctor and please get help.*

Causes of Impotence

Impotence is not something that visits you once in a blue moon; it's a consistent failure to achieve an erection stiff enough to have intercourse.

What is impotence? On the face of it, that might seem like a silly question. Actually, failing to get an erection doesn't necessarily mean you're impotent.

First of all, erections, like beauty, are in the eyes of the beholder. I see men at the Male Health Center who consider their erections to be eights and nines in terms of hardness. But when we give them injections, we find that their eights and nines are fives on our scale. Other guys take the injections and promptly declare the erection a five, when our scale rates it a ten.

Second, there might not be a man older than thirty who hasn't failed on some occasion to produce an erection. We are not robots; we are male humans who have emotions and concerns. We get tired, we get anxious, we get distracted, we get preoccupied with everyday worries. You should not expect to provide an erect penis if you're lying in bed mentally revising your company's budget projections for the next fiscal year. Impotence is not something that visits you once in a blue moon; it's a consistent failure to achieve an erection stiff enough to have intercourse.

Third, a number of drugs and medications can interfere with your erections, despite the fact that you have no physiological or psychological problem that makes you impotent. Chief among these is alcohol. It's a common misconception that a stiff drink enhances sex. Not so. Alcohol is a depressant, and taken in more than small amounts, it reduces your ability to get an erection. It also has destructive effects on your body that can cause long-term physiological difficulties with erections. Drink too much for too long, and the drinks might be the only things that are stiff.

Tobacco has both an immediate and a long-term, erection-suppressing effect. Nicotine directly interferes with the nerve pathways that produce and maintain an erection, and tobacco smoke causes heart disease and circulatory problems that can reduce the supply of blood to your penis and destroy the flexibility of tissues in the penis.

Several classes of prescription medications can hamper potency. If you're taking drugs for any of the following conditions and have developed erection problems, don't discontinue taking the drugs, but do talk to your doctor. (A detailed list of prescription drugs that have been reported to cause male problems is included in the appendix.) You should also know that potency problems with medications are not always well documented—probably because people are so reluctant to talk about failure to get an erection—so you should always talk to your doctor any time you take a new medication and have any adverse effect. Your medication might be switched or modified, and that might just solve your problems in the bedroom.

Conditions Treated With Drugs That Can Hamper Erections

- High blood pressure
- Angina
- Ulcer
- Irritable bowel syndrome
- Anxiety
- Depression
- Psychosis
- Obesity
- Heroin addiction
- Alcohol addiction
- Tuberculosis

- **Insomnia**
- **Prostate cancer**
- **Glaucoma**

> *The message here is not to stop taking your medication when you think you have a problem. See your doctor and talk to him.*

In many cases, when you stop taking a drug that has been getting in the way of your sex life, you get better—although it's certainly possible that the condition for which the drug was prescribed is also hampering your sexual enjoyment. Among the prescription drugs, switching to another might produce a quick response. It might take longer, however, to see improvement when you stop drinking excessively or give up tobacco, and you might never get all the way back where you once were. But even smokers and drinkers who clean up their acts see marked improvement in both their sexual function and their health overall. And it's never too late. Recoveries have been documented into the eighth decade of life.

An example? A man came to see me for problems with erections. He had been on anti-ulcer medication for some time. We talked about the possible connection between his problem and his pills. His doctor changed his medication, and…voila!…he was able to function again.

The message here is *not* to stop taking your medication when you think you have a problem. See your doctor and talk to him.

Diseases that Cause Impotence

The physical problems that make men impotent also happen to be the most common diseases that kill them: high blood pressure, high cholesterol, and diabetes. (We diagnose one or two cases of diabetes each month at the Male Health Center.) All three contribute to the breakdown of your circulatory system, damaging arteries that supply your penis and the tiny blood vessels and blood-vessel tissue inside the penis itself. If you've got one of these problems, it's like grounding out to the second baseman. But if you've got all three, you're hitting into a triple play—big trouble.

That's why impotence should be considered a symptom of other problems. Of the men who come to the Male Health Center with potency problems, 25 percent have high cholesterol, 50 percent smoke, and many have high blood pressure. As I mentioned before, I often find myself telling a man that we can restore his erections—but he might not be around to enjoy them.

Although it's probably the most common cause of impotence, many people fail to think of arteriosclerosis (hardening and clogging of the arteries) as a disease. More commonly, it's called heart disease, because damaged heart arteries can be a very significant problem. But remember that the penis might have the highest concentration of blood vessels and blood-vessel tissue in the body. Because the penis is usually smaller than the heart (although some guys are reluctant to admit it!), its blood vessels are more easily plugged. Cholesterol also has a direct destructive effect on the spongy tissue in the penis.

As I mentioned in the symptoms section of Step One, loss of erections is often the first clear sign of a more serious illness. A study at UCLA (University of California at Los Angeles) has shown that 25 percent of men who are diagnosed as being impotent because of blood-vessel problems have a heart attack or stroke within five years.

Estimates are that over half of all men who develop diabetes as adults suffer from erection problems. Diabetes attacks potency in two ways: First, it worsens the progression of heart disease, increasing blood-supply problems for the penis. And second, it causes degeneration of the nerves that control erections. It's not as hopeless as it sounds. By reading Step Five, you already know that many (if not most) cases of adult

> *Because the penis is usually smaller than the heart (although some guys are reluctant to admit it!), its blood vessels are more easily plugged. Cholesterol also has a direct destructive effect on the spongy tissue in the penis.*

diabetes can be avoided (or even reversed) by proper diet and exercise.

A variety of less common problems can cause impotence. Multiple sclerosis, although less common than diabetes, might be even more likely to cause potency problems. MS, as it's called, is a neurological disorder that causes weakness, fatigue, difficulty in movement, and spasms. It typically strikes between the ages of twenty and forty, and studies have shown that between two-thirds and three-quarters of the men who get MS have sexual problems. Strokes, nerve damage from alcoholism, paralysis from accidents, Parkinson's disease, surgery, and even spinal disk problems can cause impotence as well.

Under the Knife

Then, too, there are occasional impotence problems caused by surgical complications when the nerves taking the messages to the blood vessels are actually cut. I saw one man, thirty-four, who had undergone three surgeries in six months for a bowel disorder and had lost his ability to get erections. Another man had prostate cancer surgery and couldn't get erect; he's very worried about it, and the sad fact is he might never be able to get natural erections again. It's not uncommon for nerves to be cut during prostate cancer surgery, leading to irreversible problems.

On the brighter side, I recently saw a man six weeks after he had radical prostate cancer surgery. He told me that he had already had sexual relations and had ejaculated. That's the record, as far as I know.

Why Things Go Wrong

Blood Supply

Let's talk about why an erection fails to happen so you can see how significant the condition of your circulatory system can be. What happens if the arteries supplying blood to the lower half of your body get clogged up and stiff? The available flow will be less than ideal for filling the penis, and there will be less blood pressure to squeeze those veins closed against the tunica albuginea. (Remember the flexible covering around the penis?)

Often, a man will be able to get a good erection, but when he begins thrusting, his legs and buttocks need blood for their muscles, and the supply gets routed away (what we doctors call a steal). And arterial problems can ruin erections in other ways. When you eat a fatty diet, get high cholesterol, and smoke cigarettes, those harmful byproducts circulate in your system, doing damage. The smaller arteries inside your penis shrink and lose their flexibility, as do the lakes that fill inside the cavities, and they won't respond as they should. Your supply and storage are affected at the same time.

> *When you eat a fatty diet, get high cholesterol, and smoke cigarettes, those harmful byproducts circulate in your system, doing damage.*

As you can begin to see, although we can talk about two different types of flow problems that can disrupt erections—poor inflow and inability to stop outflow—they actually go hand in hand. Without good inflow, it's not easy to stop the outflow. In fact, I rarely find an impotent man who has only one of these problems.

But there is still an important distinction between inflow and outflow problems. An inflow problem can be corrected if you suffer from it; but problems with outflow cannot be corrected, only prevented. Research by Dean Ornish has shown that a very low-fat diet, exercise, and mental relaxation can actually reverse the accumulation of plaque in arteries. So inflow problems that are a result of arteriosclerosis can be improved by changing your life-style.

Outflow problems, however, might be a result of irreversible damage to the tissue in the cavities. Urological researchers led by Dr. Goldstein believe that the spongy tissue inside the penis actually breaks down—probably because of poor life-style, but genetics might play a role, too—and becomes incapable of expanding and storing blood. No one knows how to rejuvenate this tissue, so proper maintenance is vital, or you'll have to resort to artificial means of getting an erection.

When Your Mind Is Not Your Ally

As I said back in the beginning of this step, although physiological problems might be at the root of most cases of impotence, no man has an erection problem without having a psychological problem. Men who physiologically might be able to have sex, can't. And sometimes, just one failure (maybe because he's had too much to drink) can saddle a man with what is really a psychological case of impotence. Here's how:

Have you ever been startled while you had an erection? Did you notice how quickly that erection went away? Our bodies have evolved over tens of thousands of years not to have erections when we're frightened. We don't want an erection when we're cheering at a football game, caught in the middle of an argument, or being robbed. When we get excited or scared, our nervous systems move blood away from nonessential activities and into muscles so we can either fight or flee. Our nerves release adrenaline called norepinephrine, which stops an erection immediately. Norepinephrine doesn't exist only in mass quantities, producing that intense surge you feel when someone leaps around a corner. It seeps into your system and is released into the penis any time you're anxious.

I can't emphasize too much how powerful an influence the mind can be on your potency or lack of same. Think of it as the equivalent of a set of weights hanging from the end of the penis. Maybe there's a little bit of an inflow restriction and little bit of an outflow problem. Together, they're not enough to hold the penis down. But add a little worry about performing—maybe the result of only one fading erection—and the adrenaline is

> *Our bodies have evolved over tens of thousands of years not to have erections when we're frightened. We don't want an erection when we're cheering at a football game, caught in the middle of an argument, or being robbed. When we get excited or scared, our nervous systems move blood away from nonessential activities and into muscles so we can either fight or flee.*

enough to tip the scales and ruin your evening. Your doctor could call it vascular (circulatory) impotence or psychogenic (psychological) impotence, but it's really both at the same time. The important thing is to do what's most practical to treat either or both, and lift off some of that weight.

It's also important to understand that you can become conditioned to respond this way, so that you don't even notice that a sexual situation makes you nervous. For example, you realize there is a chance you will have sex that night. You worry about being able to function, and the result is anxiety. Then here comes the norepinephrine to douse your erection. After the experience has been repeated a number of times, it becomes automatic. You need to unlearn that response and learn a new one.

Figuring out What's Gone Wrong

Your urologist—the specialist who diagnoses and treats impotence—has an impressive array of equipment to test for different causes of a potency problem, but most of it is seldom necessary. That's because finding the absolute cause of a potency problem isn't always necessary or even desirable. We have to find a balance that works for the patient. For a seventy-year-old man, the important thing is just to get him functioning. For a thirty-five-year-old, it's more important to find the precise cause. Frankly, a label doesn't do you a heck of a lot of good in the bedroom, and the treatment might be the same regardless of the root cause.

Sometimes, a cure can be found through a sit-down visit with your doctor to discuss what has happened. Your doctor should review all the medications you've been taking, ask about your drinking habits, and request a full medical history—of events related to your problem and those that might seem unconnected. There's a chance that a simple change of medication, or some change in your diet or drinking habits, will help you get back in line.

> *We typically diagnose prostate cancer in five to ten men a year who come in to see us with erection problems.*

When a man is having problems with potency, certain parts of an examination should be standard. At the Male Health Center, we routinely take your blood pressure, conduct a testicle exam (for shriveling and for cancer) and do a prostate exam. We typically diagnose prostate cancer in five to ten men a year who come in to see us with erection problems. More extensive testing can include blood work that measures both total and free testosterone (the active component of the hormone), although low hormone levels probably cause less than 10 percent of erection difficulties. Other blood tests can turn up problems such as diabetes, high cholesterol, and thyroid conditions.

Depending on your age and physical condition, you might have some tests to check your nerve function. Some of these are as simple as pin pricks or response to a vibrating tuning fork. The bulbocavernosal reflex, which contracts the rectum when the head of the penis is squeezed—I assure my patients I'm not getting fresh—is another clue to proper nerve operation. Biothesiometry, where a vibration is applied to the penis by what is, in effect, an electrical tuning fork, measures the threshold of sensation, which is an important part of getting an erection. We also check pulse and blood pressure in the penis, although it's not clear how accurate penile blood pressure is. At the same time, the doctor should examine the penis for plaques that might be a sign of Peyronie's disease (more about that later).

Many urologists are finding the erection injection to be one of the most effective tools in diagnosing potency problems. I use a substance that occurs naturally in the body, called prostaglandin E1 (PGE), which is injected through a *tiny* needle (producing next to no pain—honest, guys). Acting much like the nitric oxide, it relaxes smooth muscles in the penis to produce an erection in most men within ten minutes. The quality of that erection (remember the one-to-ten scale?) tells a lot about inflow

After some instruction on the use of the injections, a little field testing at home—where patients are much more likely to respond—can be helpful.

problems, and its duration tells a lot about outflow problems.

Many guys, however, get so anxious at the thought of a needle and are so distracted by the medical office environment, that not even PGE will overcome the adrenaline running around in their bodies. After some instruction on the use of the injections, a little field testing at home—where patients are much more likely to respond—can be helpful. Some patients who drive in from distant cities will bring their partners and check into a hotel room. We show them how to use the injection and let them try it out there, so we can monitor the duration of the erection.

Back in Step One, I mentioned a self-test for potency problems—the postage stamp test. It indicates whether a man is having normal erections during the night, while he sleeps. Doctors have somewhat more sophisticated tools to do essentially the same job. A snap gauge, which consists of several strings of various strengths, gives more than a yes-or-no idea of nighttime activity. There are also electronic recording devices for detecting nocturnal penile tumescence (NPT) to accomplish this, but the cost is justified by the additional information they offer only in certain cases.

When a man turns out to have a blood-flow problem, the urologist might perform some additional tests to figure out the exact cause. Doppler ultrasound allows us to measure the blood-flow response in the penis and the size of the arteries; by giving an erection injection, we can see if the flow increases to certain levels and also if there are leaks.

Blood flow through the penis can also be checked by dynamic infusion cavernosometry and cavernosography (DICC), which can be performed at a hospital on an outpatient basis. From this test, the doctor can determine the exact blood pressure in the penis, the rate of flow in and out, and just which vessels might be leaking. Most men won't ever need DICC, but you should never submit to vascular surgery without first going through it. (We'll talk below about more things you should do before resorting to such extremes.)

I urge every man who sees me for a potency problem to see a psychologist I practice with. As I've already said, most potency problems might not be psychological at their roots, but 100 percent of men with potency problems have an emotional problem as a result. If at all possible, the partner should be included. Impotence is not just a man's disease. It affects the partner, as well. And it usually takes both working together to solve the problem.

Impotence is not just a man's disease. It affects the partner, as well. And it usually takes both working together to solve the problem.

In the 90s, There's No Reason Not to Have an Erection

Sexual Healing

There are five vitally important things for you to remember when seeking treatment for impotence:

1 Every problem can be treated; impotence is not something you have to live with.

2 It's not often necessary to completely eliminate all the problems that cause impotence. Remember, the penis can be like a set of scales loaded down with various weights. Take a few out and the balance will shift.

3 There are always treatment options; there is never only one best treatment.

4 Consider the psychological factors.

5 Don't forget the partner.

The most sensible approach is to try the simplest, least-invasive techniques first, assuming that those are acceptable to the patient. So the following treatments are listed in rough order of their ease, expense, and irreversibility. Remember that all these treatments are aimed toward getting the penis hard. Orgasm and ejaculation are separate events, and these treatments should make both possible.

**Pelvic Floor
Biofeedback**

Although the muscles *inside* your penis must relax in order for you to have an erection, muscles outside the penis, but mostly inside your body—the ones that contract to make you ejaculate—must be tensed to help erections. (You might want to look back at Figure 3 on page 144). We've known for some time that when the muscles called ischiocavernosus (IC) and bulbovaernosus (BC) contract, blood pressure inside the penis increases significantly, stiffening the erection. Usually, these muscles operate without any conscious thought on your part, but it occurred to a group of Belgian researchers that men might be taught to use and strengthen the IC muscle to improve erections that were not stiff enough for intercourse.

This is a very new approach, and no one knows for sure just how successful it will turn out to be. However, I'm beginning to see reports in the literature of pelvic floor exercises producing good results. We're beginning to utilize it at the Male Health Center and are encouraged because the technique is so noninvasive. The procedure is much like the Kegel exercise—a tensing of the pelvic floor that many women do to maintain good muscle tone in their pelvic area—but techniques are used to teach men how to accentuate the IC muscle. The Belgians used electrical stimulation to contract the IC muscle, so that the men would know what contraction of the proper muscle felt like. It's also possible to apply sensors that let a man know, when he's tensing the right muscle (called biofeedback).

The Belgians used this approach in an attempt to improve the rigidity of men's erections. After four months of pelvic exercise training, sixty-nine out of 155 men were cured, and another forty-two had improved. Early results at my clinic have not been quite so encouraging, but I think the approach is worth pursuing further. And in any event, better pelvic floor fitness benefits men as well as women. You'll hear more about it later in this step.

Oral Medications

In any event, yohimbine causes few side effects in most people (occasional jitters and blood pressure increase in some), and it's not very expensive.

No one knows if yohimbine just has a psychological (placebo) effect—or, if it is physiological, whether it works in the brain or penis— but if the effect is psychological, this case shows once more just how powerful the mind can be.

The drug yohimbine, prepared from the bark of an African tree called yohimbe, has been touted for its enhancement of both sexual desire and erections for decades. Until recently, however, there was little solid scientific research to support its use. Two studies published in 1989 (both supported by pharmaceutical companies), suggest that yohimbine might be of real help to somewhere between 20 and 40 percent of men.

In any event, yohimbine causes few side effects in most people (occasional jitters and blood pressure increase in some), and it's not very expensive. (However, a study done by *Men's Confidential* newsletter found that over-the-counter yohimbine products were inconsistent in their dosages and no less expensive than prescription preparations.) The only real disadvantages to its use are that you need to take it three times per day, and improvement doesn't usually occur for at least two weeks. Yohimbine is a good way to start the treatment of a potency problem, and it might be especially helpful for men who don't have advanced physical causes for their problem.

I recently prescribed yohimbine for a man who'd been having erection difficulties. He returned to the Male Health Center after two months and reported that he had had sex thirty times in the previous six weeks. No one knows if yohimbine just has a psychological (placebo) effect—or, if it is physiological, whether it works in the brain or penis—but if the effect is psychological, this case shows once more just how powerful the mind can be.

Another medication that might help some men is Trental [pentoxifylline], which reduces the thickness of blood, thus increasing flow. The time-release version of this medication has minimal side effects, so if you have a blood-supply problem, you might consider discussing its use with your doctor.

Finally, the side effects of Trazodone (also called Desyrel)—one of the antidepressant medications— have helped restore sex drive in some men. It appears that it might work synergistically with yohimbine to increase libido. Using a drug for its side effects, however, is a questionable business: Another of this drug's side effects appears to be retrograde (into the bladder) ejaculation.

Maybe It's the Medicine, Man

If you're supposed to take medicine regularly, make a real effort to stay with it. Sure, popping those pills on time can be inconvenient, especially when you're traveling and you're tired at the end of the day. Certain side effects (and all medications have potential side effects) can make you wonder if the whole thing is worthwhile.

Case in point: A minister came to see me with a two-year history of problems with erections. We talked, and lo and behold, I found he was on blood-pressure medicine.

I said, "Reverend, how long have you had the problem with erections?"

"Two years," he replied.

"And how long have you been on the blood-pressure medicine?"

"Two years."

The point is to talk with your doctor. Never hesitate to let him know if you're uncomfortable.

Nobody had warned him that certain blood-pressure medicines can interfere with sexual function. It wasn't my place to change his medicine, but I advised him to go back to his doctor and tell him about the problem. He did, and I got a note from him a few weeks later saying everything was fine. His doctor had tried a different medication, and he was functioning again. But he had suffered needlessly for two years, and there are plenty more guys out there like him. Don't you be one.

The point here is not to get paranoid about all medicines. The point is to talk with your doctor. Never hesitate to let him know if you're uncomfortable. Don't be one of the more than 50 percent of patients who, studies show, "forget" or simply don't take their medicine as prescribed. That defeats the purpose, wastes your money, delays your getting well, and allows such problems as high cholesterol and high blood pressure to produce more serious effects.

Hormone Supplements

One of the most common misconceptions about impotence is that it is often caused by low levels of sex hormones. The fact is, however, that inadequate testosterone is very rarely *the* cause. It might be a contributing factor, especially in older men, but there is usually some other psycho-physiological basis for an inability to get or stay erect. A simple shot of testosterone won't often do the job. Back in the fifties and early sixties, it was all we had, and it rarely worked.

Useful levels of the male hormone do decline as we age—perhaps as much as 40 percent between about age fifty and seventy—not because we produce so much less, but because a blood protein makes some of it useless. What the full significance of having less useful testosterone might be, however, we don't really know. But it's clear that hormones are a part of a complex of factors that bring about or are a result of aging—what has been called male menopause or "viropause" in Europe.

It's a subject few people know much about, but it should get widespread exposure in an upcoming book by Gail Sheehy. Sheehy, the author of *Silent Passage*, a book about female menopause, is now working on a sequel about what happens to men as they age. In my own practice, I've had the opportunity to review the literature on the subject, and have worked closely with Gail Sheehy. In fact, she visited the Male Health Center in July 1993 to interview men about "the unspeakable passage."

Men clearly do not go through any abrupt physiological change comparable to the complete shutdown of a woman's ovaries at menopause, but we do go through significant changes. Along with a gradual decrease in testosterone levels, we tend to lose muscle mass, our blood slows, the velocity of

Along with a gradual decrease in testosterone levels, we tend to lose muscle mass, our blood slows, the velocity of nerve transmissions decreases, and our attitude and aggressiveness change.

nerve transmissions decreases, and our attitude and aggressiveness change.

The issues raised by male hormonal decline are complicated and thorny. Some European doctors advocate giving older men testosterone supplements, much the way postmenopausal women are sometimes given estrogen. The theory is that older men who get testosterone supplements will maintain more muscle mass, have stronger bones, gain less weight, and suffer less from depression—not to mention having a strong interest in sex. And there's no question that men who have levels on the low side feel happier and more energetic when given supplements.

Sounds pretty good, until you hear about the potential down side. There is strong evidence that the prostate—the gland that produces the bulk of semen—responds to testosterone levels. Testosterone might cause the prostate to grow larger—potentially causing urination problems—and eliminating it from the body curbs the growth rate of prostate cancers. (From that, we infer that testosterone plays a role in prostate cancer growth, but there is no convincing evidence that high testosterone levels predispose a man to developing prostate cancer.) It appears that taking supplemental testosterone can be much like pouring gasoline on a fire.

In addition, hormones can cause liver damage and, in rare cases, liver cancer. They thicken the blood, increasing the risk of circulatory problems. And they reduce the body's ability to produce its own hormones, resulting in lifetime dependency.

The upshot? I think that testosterone supplementation is far too simplistic an approach to treating erection problems—let alone aging. We need to deal with the whole man—his diet and exercise habits, his other physiological problems, his relationship with his partner, his ability to communicate, and, indeed, sometimes his hormone levels. A man might need some additional testosterone, but only as a part of an overall approach to improving his health and

> *We need to deal with the whole man—his diet and exercise habits, his other physiological problems, his relationship with his partner, his ability to communicate, and, indeed, sometimes his hormone levels.*

Part of the problem with testosterone supple-mentation today is that injections are the only practical way to administer it, but they result in a rapid increase and then decrease in blood levels.

life. And if he does get testosterone, he needs to be monitored closely for prostate cancer.

My hesitancy about testosterone supplementation is based on experience. At the Male Health Center, we have been treating a man who was given testosterone shots by another doctor for two years. The shots did nothing to solve his potency problem, and he came to us because he was having difficulty urinating. We diagnosed very advanced (incurable) prostate cancer—and ironically, the supplements weren't even helping him.

Part of the problem with testosterone supplementation today is that injections are the only practical way to administer it, but they result in a rapid increase and then decrease in blood levels. Oral preparations are metabolized in the liver, reducing their effect significantly. In the future, patches that adhere to the skin might help solve these problems.

I have a simple prescription for testosterone, however. Most research has shown that men who get regular, moderate aerobic exercise—see the recommendations in Step Four—have higher testosterone levels, both while they exercise and in between exercise sessions. (Don't overdo it, though; highly trained endurance athletes might actually have lower testosterone levels.) So testosterone response might be at least one of the reasons why regular exercisers have less depression, more libido, and a happier sex life. For the time being, then, stay away from testosterone supplements unless a blood test shows that your level is truly low. Instead, make your own hormone by working out.

Vacuum Devices

This is the least invasive—although not necessarily the least expensive or obtrusive—form of impotence treatment. Consisting of a plastic cylinder that fits snugly over the penis and is sealed to the body with water-based jelly, and a vacuum pump, the device produces negative pressure around the penis, causing blood to flow in. Usually, once an erection has been established, an elastic ring slips onto the base of the penis to hold blood in, allowing the tube to be removed. In fact, some men find they need only the rings to retain an erection they were able to achieve naturally (Figure 7).

Vacuum Erection Device: *Figure 7*

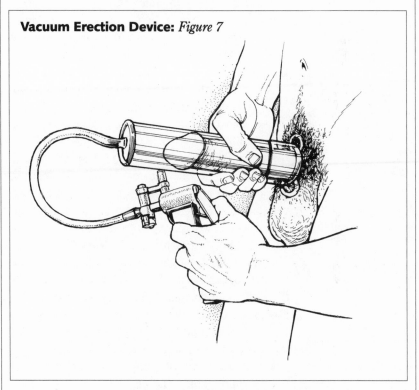

If a vacuum device is used properly—instruction is important—it will produce an erection in just about any man. (They have been used successfully on paralyzed men, who have no sensation in their penis.) Because the erection is being maintained by a constriction ring at the base of the penis, the portion of the penis inside the body might not be as rigid, producing a hinge effect. The skin temperature of the penis might also be somewhat colder than normal, because of the flow restriction. What's more, the constriction ring must not be left on for longer than thirty minutes, lest damage occur.

Remember, it takes time and practice to get good at using a vacuum.... I encourage everyone with erection problems to at least try a vacuum device.

Those minor disadvantages aside, vacuum devices are well accepted by many men and nearly all women. Although they require some planning and preparation for sex, they are effective and have no side effects. Some men discover that after using a vacuum device for a while, they're able to get an erection without the device. This could be because of the restorative effects of pulling fresh, oxygenated blood into the penis, or it could be because of the confidence built by knowing you can have an erection. Most likely, it's a combination of the two.

You should obtain vacuum devices through your doctor (most, but not all, manufacturers require a prescription)—to be sure you get a quality device that's the right size and get proper instruction (videos are available for you to take home). Remember, it takes time and practice to get good at using a vacuum. You can expect to pay between $200 and $400 (avoid those cheap substitutes in the magazine ads), but most urologists will be willing to loan you one—the Male Health Center has one of the largest collections in Texas—so you can see if it's the right solution. I encourage everyone with erection problems to at least try a vacuum device.

Not every couple can accept the fact that applying a vacuum device requires either planning or a pause in sexual activity (and it's definitely not for the guy who's looking for fast love in a singles bar), but many find it a perfectly satisfactory and safe way to enjoy sex again. One man was so enthusiastic about the unit we loaned him that he refused to return it until his prescription-ordered vacuum device arrived. Another man, a salesman in his sixties, found that the vacuum worked very well for him. Now his wife says she'll worry if she ever sees him packing the vacuum to take on a trip.

Erection Injections

About 80 percent of all men with a potency problem respond to an injection of prostaglandin E1 or a combination of prostaglandin E1, papaverine, and

Another man, a salesman in his sixties, found that the vacuum worked very well for him. Now his wife says she'll worry if she ever sees him packing the vacuum to take on a trip.

Once a man has had his first injection in the office, it's not uncommon for him to ask for a gallon of it to go.

phentolamine—all drugs that relax smooth muscle in the penis. The drugs work just like the nitric oxide in the penis—letting the blood flow in and not get out.

The needle is the tiniest made, and it is inserted in an area with very few nerve endings. Although any sensible man would be apprehensive before his first injection, most find that it's not uncomfortable. It requires some instruction, but it's not difficult to do. Within five to ten minutes, he gets an erection on the eight-to-ten scale that lasts thirty to sixty minutes, and even after ejaculation, the erection might not go away until the drug fades.

Once a man has had his first injection in the office, it's not uncommon for him to ask for a gallon of it to go. One guy, however, got an injection and didn't make it home to enjoy it. He had a flat tire (a real one) in the middle of rush-hour traffic, full erection and all. There will be no jokes about tire tools.

None of the medications currently used for erection injections are approved by the Food and Drug Administration (FDA), but all of the previously mentioned medications have been proved safe in other applications and have been used for erection help for most of a decade. There are also new compounds being developed that will be released in the not-too-distant future.

The primary side effect of Prostaglandin E1, a naturally occurring compound in the body, is a burning sensation after injection. This has recently been shown to be a result of the acidity of the medicines. Buffering them with sodium bicarbonate appears to eliminate this problem. There have also been reports of scarring and nodules (Peyronie's disease, which we'll talk about in detail shortly)—but mainly with papaverine used alone, which is an approach that's out of favor in the medical community.

An erection that won't go away (priapism) is always a risk with injections—especially early on when we're trying to establish the correct dosage.

I try to keep my patients' erections under two hours, which takes some fine-tuning. Any erection that lasts longer than three or four hours requires immediate medical attention to prevent damage to the penis. The never-ending erection might sound like a dream come true, but it can get old.

Injections aren't for everyone, but many men find them to be a very acceptable way to get and maintain an erection. Studies have shown that quite often, men without major physical problems return to normal erections after using injections for a while.

One man who has been quite satisfied with injection therapy originally came to me after he suffered damage to the nerves that control erection during an emergency abdominal surgery. He'd been unable to have an erection for seven years and had simply given up on sex, losing his marriage along the way. In my office, he responded immediately to prostaglandin E1, and his first question to the nurse on hand was, "How often can I use this stuff?" (About three times a week is the answer.) Sporting an erection that he called "a twelve on a scale of ten," he had a second question: "Where's the phone? I want to call my girlfriend."

He'd been unable to have an erection for seven years and had simply given up on sex, losing his marriage along the way. . . . he responded immediately to prostaglandin E1, and his first question to the nurse on hand was, "How often can I use this stuff?"

He's now a strong advocate for erection injections, and, at sixty-one, he's about to remarry. "I've been on injection therapy for three years," he says. "It is flawless, and there are no side effects. It's very, very easy to do. Within five or six minutes it's there, as big as I've ever had, and I know it's going to be there. It works."

There are now ongoing studies using topical creams that are applied to the penis in an effort to produce erections without using needles. These are in the preliminary stages, and I hope to be involved in some of these investigative studies.

Vascular Surgery

When the less-invasive options fail, it's time to consider surgical correction. A few years ago, many urologists and patients opted for vascular surgery,

> *There are still times when vascular surgery is called for, but you should be very sure that yours is one of them.*

in which arteries and/or veins are rearranged or blocked off to solve inflow or outflow problems. Now, however, these approaches are less in favor because we've learned that few patients are really well suited for it. Typically, when a man has arterial problems, all his arteries, blood vessels, and the spongy tissue of the penis are affected, so patching a few vessels doesn't do the job. But even in ideal candidates—young men who have been injured, perhaps by straddling a fence, or being kicked— the success rate is only about 60 percent.

So vascular surgery isn't the solution unless specific flow problems—rather than general inability to block outflow—can be identified. There are still times when vascular surgery is called for, but you should be very sure that yours is one of them. This is a case where you should never proceed without at least a second opinion—and not just any urologist should be doing the work. Seek out an experienced, skilled surgeon at a university medical center or in a practice that specializes in potency treatments and vascular surgery.

After casting all that doubt on vascular surgery, I think it's worth mentioning that it can be very successful. I treated one eighteen-year-old man who came to me when considering marriage. He had never been able to have an erection and wanted to know if there was any way he could consummate his marriage if he were to go ahead. We were able to find specific vein leaks using DICC. He opted for surgery, and six weeks later he was married and able to function. I got a note from him two years after that saying that everything was fine, and that he and his wife had just had their first child.

Penile Implants

When a man can't or won't succeed with other treatments, an implant is the last resort. Of all the approaches, this one carries the most irrevocable consequences. Once you've had an implant, that's it— the normal spongy tissue has been damaged and

One of the saddest things I see in my practice is when a man has had an implant that he didn't really need, but was sold one anyway.

destroyed, and your chances of ever functioning normally again are gone. Implants can be removed, but normal erections will not be possible. At best, an erection will be possible only with a vacuum device in some cases. One of the saddest things I see in my practice is when a man has had an implant that he didn't really need, but was sold one anyway. Again, get at least a second opinion before considering an implant, and select your surgeon carefully. Ask about his or her experience and rate of success.

With those warnings, let me say that just because an implant is the last resort doesn't mean it's not a good one. About ten thousand penile implants are done each year, and it is my experience that many of these men—and their spouses—are delighted with the result. It's not like being eighteen again, but it's far better than nothing—the difference between having and not having intercourse. He will have the same sensation—good if it was, not so good if it wasn't—and he will be able to ejaculate normally if he was able to before.

Penile prostheses have been around for more than twenty years. Before Dr. Brantley Scott from Houston pioneered the bionics for the first implant, doctors used to implant bones under the skin of the penis. Thankfully, modern implants are both easier to install and more effective.

My first implant surgery took two and a half hours; today it takes me only fifty minutes, and it's an outpatient procedure. Early implants were semirigid—they consisted of wires coated in plastic that could be bent up for erection and more or less down for a semiflaccid condition (about a four or five on our scale). These devices are still available today. They're comparatively inexpensive, and they are durable. The next step up is the self-contained implant, a device that inflates with a fluid, but that is contained entirely within the penis. These, too, are reliable and a little more effective than a semirigid implant, yielding about a six or seven.

Today's state-of-the-art implant—what I call the Cadillac (Figure 8)—is the three-piece hydraulic implant, with a reservoir located in the abdomen for inflation. Or, if you'd rather your partner not know you're packing the pump, it can be placed behind a testicle where a woman won't notice it. These new implants achieve much more natural erect and flaccid states; they usually produce erection of eight to nine variety. In fact, one design now extends in length as it inflates. (Most implants make the penis stiff, but do not cause it to elongate or expand as much in diameter as a natural erection.) Most of my patients opt for the three-piece devices because they work so much better.

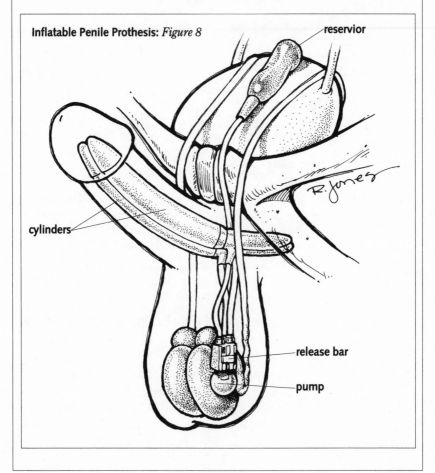

Inflatable Penile Prothesis: *Figure 8*

reservoir

cylinders

release bar

pump

During 1993, the FDA began investigating penile implants both to see just how well they're working and to look for any problems associated with the silicone used in their manufacture. The FDA suggests that every patient be informed of the following risks (beyond inherent surgical risks) before having an implant:

INFECTION

While rare, it can be a devastating problem that usually requires removal of the device.

MIGRATION

Parts of the implant might move to other locations in the body.

SCAR TISSUE

Develops around the fluid storage chamber or pump might, in rare instances, result in spontaneous erections.

MECHANICAL MALFUNCTION

Surgery might be required and, in rare instances, might cause the penis to shorten and decrease in sensation.

IMPROPER SURGICAL TECHNIQUE

Incorrect positioning or selection of the wrong size of cylinders might cause failure.

COMPLICATIONS

Infection, chronic pain, or sensory loss can occur.

UNANSWERED QUESTIONS

There are some structural and material similarities between some inflatable penile implants and some mammary implants. Although no studies of problems with penile implants have been done, problems reportedly associated with (but not scientifically proven) silicone mammary implants include immunological diseases, such as scleroderma and rheumatoid arthritis, neurological problems, and tumors of the breast.

I agree completely that all these warnings should be offered to every potential penile implant patient, but you shouldn't get the impression that problems are common. Complication and infection rates are actually very low, and the problems that do occur are almost always a result of surgical error, lack of surgical expertise, poor patient selection, or poor patient education about alternatives.

A modern implant —when properly installed in the right patient—can work wonders. It restores a man's ability to enjoy a full relationship with his partner, making his life whole again.

Out of concern for these potential problems, I reviewed more than one hundred men in whom I've installed implants over the past five years. Ninety-five percent said they were satisfied and would do it again, and 50 percent said they would go on national television to advocate penile implants. This degree of satisfaction is, I believe, the result of proper selection and education of the men so they knew what they were getting. I encourage men to talk to other men who have had implants, so they will have reasonable expectations about what it will do for them. A modern implant—when properly installed in the right patient—can work wonders. It restores a man's ability to enjoy a full relationship with his partner, making his life whole again.

One patient at the Male Health Center told me that he had willed his body to medical science after his death—all, that is, except his implant. He told me, "Doc, I might get out of here before you, and I want to be sure I've got my implant with me when I get where I'm going."

Psychological Treatment

I've already told you that I think psychological counseling is very important when treating impotence. There is no sense treating a penis as if it's not attached to an entire man who has fears, emotions, and worries. A man should explore those feelings with his partner and the help of a skilled, professional counselor. I'm not talking about psychoanalysis. Counseling for potency patients is based on issues: Understanding how performance anxiety can destroy performance and figuring out how to control it, resolving marital issues on both sides, and sometimes even treating the depression than can lead to or be a result of potency problems. There's nothing wrong with being a male who feels. In fact, it's the way we get over the things that tear us down.

Summing up the Solutions

Because I believe that information is the best antidote to fear and self-doubt, I've given you quite a lot here. Let me sum up my philosophy of treating impotence by putting the various steps in this ranking order, ranging from the simplest to the most complicated and invasive.

1 Read <u>The New Male Sexuality</u> by Bernie Zilbergeld. One man with lung disease was having problems with erections. He read Zilbergeld's book, which advocates changing your life-style for sexual improvement. Realizing he was overtired, he began taking afternoon naps. His wife joined him, he began having erections, and soon they were enjoying orgasms in the middle of the day. He was cured.

2 Get a good physical examination to check for other medical problems.

3 If you're on medication, check with your doctor to see if any changes are in order.

4 Ask about pelvic floor exercises

5 Trial doses of yohimbine

6 Vacuum

7 Penile Injections

8 Revascularization surgery, if you're an ideal candidate

9 As a last resort, the penile implant

> *The curve can be so extreme the penis forms a J or corkscrew, making intercourse impossible.*

Peyronie's Disease—A Turn for the Worse

Peyronie's disease (severe curvature of the erect penis) is a fairly common, but rarely mentioned problem. I see anywhere from five to ten men a week that have it. A minor bend in a man's penis is perfectly normal; few are arrow straight. But with Peyronie's disease, named after the physician to King Louis XIV of France (the physician who first noted the disorder back in the 1700s), the curve can be so extreme the penis forms a J or corkscrew, making intercourse impossible.

Safe sex means not only preventing sexually transmitted diseases, but practicing defensive sex as well.

Of course, for a man who gets Peyronie's, it's much worse than just a physical inability to have sex. In my observation, a man whose penis is deformed might be even more emotionally devastated than a man whose penis just won't work. First off, he needs to be assured that he does not have cancer. Then we can go on to do what can be done to get him back on the straight and narrow.

The cause of Peyronie's disease is unknown. I've seen articles suggesting that acrobatic sex, in which the penis can get bent back on itself, and even minor blows to the penis might be a factor in some cases. If that's the case, then safe sex means not only preventing sexually transmitted diseases, but practicing defensive sex as well. On the other hand, some researchers have theorized that the plaques might form as a result of the body's immune system (the system that fights disease) overreacting. There also have been reports that some men who take beta-blocking medications for high blood pressure develop Peyronie's.

The disease starts as a small bump or constriction on the shaft of the penis below the skin, which expands to form a flat deposit that's sometimes as large as the diameter of a silver dollar. This "plaque" invades and replaces the elastic covering (tunica) of the penis with inflexible material (refer back to Figure 3 on page 144). When a man with Peyronie's has an erection, the plaque does not expand, so his penis bends to one side. About one-third of men with Peyronie's have painful erections, and a few become impotent. In some cases, the head of the penis does not fill with blood. One center reports that about one in twenty-five men who make appointments for potency problems have Peyronie's disease. Dr. Irwin Goldstein has shown that the inflexibility can interfere with blocking of outflow from the penis. Other than that, however, complications are very rare.

The first step in treating Peyronie's is to be patient and see if it corrects itself. As many as one-third of these cases get better within the eighteen months after the onset of the problem, without extensive treatment.

The first step in treating Peyronie's is to be patient and see if it corrects itself. As many as one-third of these cases get better within the eighteen months after the onset of the problem, without extensive treatment. During this time, most urologists recommend taking four hundred international units of vitamin E three times a day for the disease. Reports of benefits from vitamin E come from patients, rather than medical trials, but at the very least vitamin E won't hurt you. (And it might have a protective effect against heart disease.) No other effective nonsurgical treatment exists. Steer clear of any doctor who recommends steroid injections, which don't help and might be harmful; ultrasound, which is just plain ineffective; or oral potaba, which must be taken in huge quantities (twenty-four pills per day).

Even in cases where the plaque doesn't disappear on its own within a year or two, further treatment might not be necessary. As long as the bend isn't severe enough to prevent intercourse and the problem doesn't threaten potency, many men (and their partners) learn to live with the mild curvature.

When Peyronie's doesn't improve spontaneously and the curve is so extreme that it prevents sex or affects potency, surgical correction is possible. In the hands of a skilled surgeon, the shaft of the penis can be straightened by:

1 cutting away the plaque and grafting

2 taking a tuck on the side opposite the plaque

3 installing a penile implant.

The first two approaches can result in impotence, since cutting away the plaque can damage the tunica albuginea, resulting in leaks, or the nerves in the area, causing numbness. Once again, surgical skill is crucial. The implant is the last resort, of course, but it's the best when other problems, such as impotence, are present.

Researchers from the University of California School of Medicine at San Francisco, and the

> *Nothing that affects the organ a man is most proud of can be a physical problem alone. Talking about it helps.*

Veterans Administration Medical Center in San Francisco have recently used a laser in combination with surgical techniques to remove Peyronie's plaques without damage to the tunica. Their early results— straightening in all twelve cases and no induced problems with potency— are encouraging. The laser can be used in subtle ways to evaporate the plaque without damaging nearby tissues, which helps preserve normal erections.

Just as is the case with impotence, I think it's advisable for men with Peyronie's to have a few counseling sessions with a psychologist. Nothing that affects the organ a man is most proud of can be a physical problem alone. Talking about it helps. A urologist can reassure a man with a bent penis that he does not have penile cancer. But it takes other skills and training to help a man understand that he's not alone, that his sex life is not over, and that he can get through this tough time.

One Male Health Center patient is fifty-four years old and has had Peyronie's for seven years. His bend isn't severe enough to prevent intercourse, he can still get erections, and he and his partner are still enjoying sex. He'd like to have a straight penis, and we've discussed the alternatives and the risks involved in trying to get him one. So far, he's decided that he can live with the disease.

Jumping the Gun: Premature Ejaculation

Not long ago, I saw a very distraught young man who suffered from premature ejaculation. His wife of ten years was about to leave him, complaining that she had never been sexually satisfied, because he ejaculated most of the time before penetrating her or seconds after penetration. By applying some of the techniques we're going to discuss in this section, we were able to improve his erection and his lasting power, and save his marriage.

Premature ejaculation suffers from some of the same definition problems as impotence. Are you a premature ejaculator if you can't always wait as long as your partner would like? Is the problem all in your head? The answer is no to both questions.

Most men would like to be able to control when they ejaculate, but few always can. But don't panic: You don't have a premature ejaculation problem unless you *frequently* ejaculate before or shortly after beginning intercourse. One study claims that thirty-six million men suffer from premature ejaculation, and it's been a vexing problem for them and the physicians who've tried to treat them. A few of the things that have not been shown to be beneficial include:

- long-term psychoanalysis
- getting drunk
- using one or more condoms
- concentrating on something other than sex—such as the batting averages of the last five American League batting champions—while having intercourse
- biting one's cheek as a distraction
- frequent masturbation
- creams that numb the penis
- testosterone injections
- tranquilizers

Before you seek treatment for premature ejaculation, it's appropriate to talk to a psychologist about other conflicts that might be affecting your sexual performance.

One approach that has been used with some success should be viewed with some caution. Prozac (fluoxetine), an antidepressant medication, is known to retard ejaculation. However, using any drug for its side effects rather than it's intended purpose is a questionable approach, and Prozac might have other effects on sexual performance.

Before you seek treatment for premature ejaculation, it's appropriate to talk to a psychologist about other conflicts that might be affecting your sexual performance. It's not unusual for a man to imagine that he can solve his marital problems by being able to last longer during intercourse, but relationship problems nearly always go deeper than that. Men also can have premature ejaculation problems related to impotence. Because they're so worried about losing an erection, they rush to a climax. Again, these can be learned responses that aren't easy to erase.

Nonetheless, one of the experts in this field, Helen Singer Kaplan, M.D., Ph.D., says that premature ejaculation—although it does cause a great deal of emotional trauma—is rarely a psychological problem at root. Instead, Dr. Kaplan views it as the failure to develop full sexual sensory awareness. A man must become fully aware of the sensations he's feeling, not trying to ignore them or dull them, so that he understands his level of excitement and isn't taken by surprise when the moment of climax arrives.

Although she is a psychiatrist, Dr. Kaplan doesn't recommend intense psychological therapy to help men get control. Instead, she encourages men and their partners to talk openly about the situation—perhaps in the presence of a counselor—and practice step-by-step methods for getting control. There are two standard approaches, which achieve the same thing by slightly different means.

The Squeeze Method

This approach was developed by Masters and Johnson. The partner stimulates the man's penis until he is close to the point of ejaculation. He must tell her when he's about to ejaculate, at which point she squeezes his penis with her hand hard enough to make him partially lose his erection. (By wrapping fingers around the penis just below the head, a squeeze will efficiently prevent ejaculation.) The goal is for the man to become well enough aware of the sensations that he learns how to forestall his orgasm on his own. The technique progresses from manual stimulation to motionless intercourse with the woman on top, to her moving, to both moving.

Researchers at Masters and Johnson claim that 98 percent of couples taught these techniques by qualified sex therapists can overcome the problem.

To find a therapist, call the American Association of Sex Educators, Counselors and Therapists. (Phone number is at end of this step.)

The Stop-Start Method

This approach was first used by Dr. James Semons in 1955, and Dr. Kaplan and other therapists have refined it considerably. Dr. Kaplan describes the method in great detail in her book, *PE: How to Overcome Premature Ejaculation*, but here briefly is what's involved. (Dr. Zilbergeld's book, *The New Male Sexuality,* also discusses techniques for conquering premature ejaculation.)

Stop-start begins much like the squeeze method, except that the woman just stops stimulating the man's penis when he asks her to—before the point of inevitability. As soon as he's certain he's under control, he asks her to begin rubbing again.

This procedure is repeated three times before allowing ejaculation on the fourth. After the couple has repeated this two or three times a week and he has gained good control, stop-start with lubrication is introduced. After that has been mastered, intercourse with the woman on top and the man not moving can be attempted. Again he asks that she stop when he approaches the point of no return. That's followed by female-superior intercourse with the man moving his hips, which is followed by stop-start, side-by-side intercourse. Finally, slowing down is substituted for stopping and starting. Yes, it's a lot of work, but it has good fringe benefits. We've had several guys go through the program and they've learned to retard their ejaculation.

Using this approach, Dr. Kaplan reports being able to cure 90 percent of her patients. In my own practice, the success rate is not quite so high, largely because partners aren't always cooperative about performing all the steps. A man can practice stop-start without a partner, but the effects go only so far. For men with partners who aren't willing to participate, premature ejaculation can remain a frustrating problem. For that reason, at the Male Health Center we've been exploring new techniques to treat this problem.

Biofeedback Therapy

Based on two studies presented at a meeting of the International Society for Impotence Research in September 1992, the Male Health Center is using biofeedback to help men control ejaculation. That research demonstrated that men who ejaculate prematurely have hyperactive pelvic muscles, the ones that surround the base of the penis and contract strongly to cause ejaculation. These muscles are already on their way toward ejaculation as soon as a man with premature ejaculation becomes excited. We have also noticed during biothesiometry measurements that a man with premature ejaculation tends to have an unusually sensitive penis. Combine these two things, and a man's ballgame is going to end in the fifth inning.

> *Combine these two things, and a man's ballgame is going to end in the fifth inning.*

Biofeedback allows a man to become aware of the muscles that control ejaculation and learn how to control them. Using electrodes, a biofeedback therapist can help men identify these muscles and learn how to relax them. Thirty men have signed up for our initial study group and are going through a series of office and in-home training sessions. Response from men interested in solving their problem has been overwhelming, and the preliminary results are encouraging.

One thirty-five-year-old man, married for about ten years, had never been able to last more than ten seconds after penetration. At this writing, he had been on the program for six weeks and reported lasting twelve to fifteen minutes, and he and his wife have experienced tremendous enjoyment.

Still, regardless of the technique that is used, there is no quick fix to conquer premature ejaculation. All of these exercises require time, practice, and patience. Remember that you're trying to overcome years of conditioning. You can't run a triathlon after training for a week.

Q A MAN TO MAN

QUESTION	ANSWER
Don't some common prescription drugs affect male problems?	Yes. Over-the-counter and prescription antihistamines can bother men with prostate problems because they affect the ability to urinate. During cold season, in fact, the urology business picks up because so many men are taking antihistamines.

QUESTION	ANSWER
Why shouldn't I buy a vacuum erection device from one of the advertisements in the back of sex magazines? They're much cheaper and look much the same.	There are several good reasons to see a doctor about a vacuum device—aside from the assurance that you'll be buying quality. First, you'll get instruction in how to use it. My own experience, and research by Dr. Perry Nadig in San Antonio, has shown that people who fail with vacuum devices usually do so because of poor technique. Second, you should get a chance to borrow one and see how well it suits you before plunking down your money. Third, some of the parts used with a vacuum device—especially the constriction rings—need periodic replacement, and the companies that work by prescription are all quite helpful about this. Finally, some of the companies that produce vacuum devices are either doing or supporting important research to advance impotence treatments, not just profiting from someone else's work.

QUESTION	ANSWER
Is there anything I can do to increase the quantity of my ejaculate?	Yes, but I don't think you'll like the recommendation. If you ejaculate less often, you'll produce more on those rare occasions. Seriously, it's normal for both ejaculate volume and the force with which it's expelled to decline as a man gets older. And the best way to forestall aging is to take good care of yourself.

QUESTION	ANSWER
Are erections we have in our sleep always accompanied by erotic dreams?	Not necessarily, but they do happen during the dream phase of sleep. Although there's much we don't understand about nocturnal erections, it's clear that they are different from daytime erotic erections in some ways. I have examined men who have erections while they sleep who don't become erect with an injection. Likewise, I've seen men who have no nighttime erections but can develop one during the day with the proper stimulation.

QUESTION	ANSWER
How does the foreskin affect sensation in sex? I've heard on the one hand that men with a foreskin enjoy sex more, and on the other that they're more likely to suffer from premature ejaculation.	This is a very sensitive issue for some men. Although I'm almost certain to offend someone, I am unaware of any convincing scientific evidence that the presence of a foreskin enhances sex or leads to premature ejaculation. I think there's a risk here of becoming too absorbed in nerves and paying too little attention to emotions. As I've said, good sex isn't performance; it's *not* a matter of anatomy or mastering technique. It takes caring and sharing. That's what can overcome premature ejaculation and what makes sex worth having.

QUESTION	ANSWER
Is it normal to masturbate even when a person is involved in a monogamous relationship?	According to surveys, the majority of men continue to masturbate at least occasionally throughout their lives—no matter their marital status. (In fact, many women do, too.) So I'd say it's normal to masturbate, but I'd also say it's normal not to. It's up to you; you're the only one who knows what you need.

QUESTION	ANSWER
I've read that a nitroglycerin patch placed on a man's penis can produce an erection. Is this a good approach to solving erection problems?	Nitroglycerin, which is used in patients with heart problems, will produce erections. It is a smooth muscle relaxant, most likely because it stimulates nitric oxide in the penis. However, nitroglycerin patches are not a safe way to induce erections because they have a number of side effects, including fainting, headaches, and dangerously low blood pressure. The nitroglycerin can also be absorbed through the woman's vagina, causing headaches. I think someone eventually will develop a patch or injection that produces an erection based on nitric oxide activity, but we haven't got a safe one yet.

QUESTION	ANSWER
I'm in my early sixties and find that I sometimes don't reach orgasm easily when my partner and I have sex. Oddly enough, this seems to bother her more than it does me. Am I losing interest?	It's not at all unusual for men to have intercourse without ejaculating when they grow older. But perhaps because it was such an important thing to their husbands when they were young, some women greet this change with concern that they're becoming less exciting. Be sure your spouse knows this isn't abnormal—tell her I said so. But more important, be sure to let her know you find her at least as exciting as ever.

HOTLINES	
American Association of Sex Educators, Counselors, and Therapists	• (312) 644-0828
Impotence Anonymous	• (615) 983-6092
Impotence Institute of America	• (800) 669-1603

7

**Avoiding or
Surviving
Sexually
Transmitted
Diseases**

PLAY IT SAFE

MEN TALK: Al Luckenbill, age twenty-nine:

*G*etting genital warts has changed my life entirely. It was four years ago, and I had a regular girlfriend—but I wasn't monogamous, even though she was. When I had sex with other women, I almost always used a condom. But I guess "almost" wasn't good enough, because I got it. Telling my girlfriend was the worst thing I ever had to do. She left me immediately.

"For two years, I saw my G.P. When he said I had condyloma, that made it sound even worse. So I went every two weeks for a liquid-nitrogen treatment. The idea was to freeze the warts off. It made a mess, but it never worked for long. I spent two years with sores healing on my penis, never having sex, and in the end I still had condyloma.

"It didn't really matter that I was healing all the time, because I had no interest in sex anyway. I'd decided to give it up entirely for the rest of my life. I was really depressed, and just thinking about the possibility of giving condyloma to someone else made me literally sick to my stomach. Believe me, knowing you might be a deadly weapon is really traumatic.

"A little over a year ago, I found a specialist. The urologist told me that there was no cure, but that we could try laser treatment to remove the visible warts. On some people, they didn't come back; on others, they did. I figured it was worth a try, so I had three tries of *laser treatments.*

"They weren't too bad really—easier than the liquid nitrogen freezes in most ways. It wasn't the physical pain that bothered me; it was the psychological stress of wondering if the warts were going to come back. And, unfortunately, although the laser removed the warts in the area where they had been for the previous three years, they did come back around the edges of the treated area.

"Right now? Well, I'm putting a chemical on twice a day, three days a week for a month. It's removed the old warts, but new ones may come back. Who knows?

"Gradually, though, I'm beginning to accept it—I think because I'm finally growing up. I am beginning to understand what things really make life fulfilling. I've met a new girl who is truly wonderful and understanding. I just hope the condyloma stays in remission. You can be darn sure I'll not be catching anything else. I've learned my lesson and I'm practicing safe sex. "

In the last six steps you've learned how to get more out of life—in both years and pleasure. *This is no time to blow it!*

I have treated thousands of men for sexually transmitted diseases ranging from pubic lice to AIDS. All of them—young, old, white, black, straight, gay, sick, and scared— have two things in common.

First, almost without exception, they thought they wouldn't be the ones to catch a disease. Maybe they made just one mistake. Or maybe they figured "nice" people don't get STDs (sexually transmitted diseases). Or maybe, like Al, they believe that wearing a condom (almost) all the time is 100-percent effective prevention. I've heard many different versions of this sad story, but they all come down to "Why me?"

Second, they've learned that catching a disease through sex does much more than just make them physically ill—it attacks the very core of their being, eating away at their confidence, their sense of self, their love of life. I've seen man after man emotionally devastated by it. They feel alone, and they are certain that no one will ever love them again. Many are ready to swear off sex forever. They feel the deepest kind of confusion, and who can blame them? All of their lives, they have been taught that a man always pursues sex, the great prize. So how could sex, an activity so pleasurable and life-enhancing, bring them to physical ruin and even death? They feel betrayed by their lovers, by themselves, by life itself.

As you probably know unless you've been living on one of the moons of Saturn, getting a sexual disease these days is not just a matter of popping in for a quick shot or a prescription and then you're all better. In fact, the most common STDs today aren't curable. Once you've got them, they are part of you, something you must live with for the duration. When, like Al Luckenbill, a man grasps that reality, it's not surprising that he becomes depressed and riddled with guilt. Take my word for it, not only can a sexually transmitted disease take your life, it can also ruin what's left of it.

Few people have a real grasp of just how common sexually transmitted diseases are. In the papers, we read mostly about AIDS. Over one hundred thousand Americans have died from it and about fourteen million people worldwide are infected with HIV right now. Those are sad statistics, and I surely don't want to give the impression that they're not terribly important, but the fact is that AIDS is so far relatively hard to catch and isn't very common compared to the other sexually transmitted diseases.

You see, Al Luckenbill has lots of company. Some epidemiologists believe that more than one in four sexually active Americans—nearly fifty-six million people—have incurable sexually transmitted

> *Some epidemiologists believe that more than one in four sexually active Americans—nearly fifty-six million people—have incurable sexually transmitted diseases. Incurable means forever. One in five—some thirty-one million people—might be carrying the incurable diseases genital herpes. We just don't know, though, because not more than a third of all people at risk have ever even been tested.*

diseases. Incurable means forever. One in seven—some thirty-one million people—might be carrying the incurable diseases genital herpes. We just don't know, though, because not more than a third of all people at risk have ever even been tested.

Think about those numbers for a minute. When you sit in the stands at a ball game, the odds are that someone with herpes sat in your seat within the last seven games. You don't get herpes from sitting, of course, but that might help you grasp the enormity of the situation. Baseball, apple pie—and herpes. Or, if you think that people who go out to ball games might not be as likely as some groups to have risky sex, then think about a crowded singles bar. How many of those happy swingers are infected and don't even know it? One in four? One in three? It's an alarming picture.

Whether you're more likely to be found at the ball park or singles bar, understand that only one in three of those carrying herpes know they have it. Sound odd? How could anyone not know they have a sexually transmitted disease? Actually, it's very common. For reasons we don't fully understand, herpes affects different people to different degrees. Many people can have it (or other diseases) and notice absolutely no symptoms. Yet they can easily pass herpes on to someone whose life will be changed forever.

Although sexually transmitted diseases are most common among the young, they know no age boundaries. A middle-aged man, married or not, who is sexually active with multiple partners had better be aware of what the risks are out there today. This is not the fifties, when gonorrhea was the disease and penicillin fixed it. I've seen these diseases cross every traditional boundary of age and social class. No one is exempt.

I've seen men in my office who were on a business trip, strayed once, and now a month later have some symptoms. They're laden with guilt. I diag-

> *Whether you're more likely to be found at the ball park or singles bar, understand that only one in three of those carrying herpes know they have it.*

nose a sexually transmitted disease and treat the man. But, lo and behold, he's had relations with his wife, and now she's been exposed. Their life is now changed forever.

What Can Happen to You—And Those You Care About

Just as sexually transmitted diseases have become more common and varied, so has the potential for damage spread. Gonorrhea or syphilis caught in time were not generally major threats to health thirty years ago. Today the range of health risks is much greater. Some of the physical problems a disease can cause include:

- Death from immune system breakdown (AIDS)
- Death of newborn (herpes)
- Deterioration of internal organs (syphilis)
- Liver disease or liver cancer (hepatitis)
- Cancers of the penis and female reproductive organs (several)
- Mental illness (syphilis)
- Sterility, female or male (several)
- Miscarriage or premature birth (ureaplasma)
- Scarring or narrowing of the urethra (several)
- Prostate inflammation or infection (several)
- Epididymal (a part of the reproductive tract) infection (several)
- Diseases of the joints (ureaplasma)

How It Catches You

All STDs other than pubic lice are transmitted by contact that allows microorganisms from one person's body to enter the other's body in one or more of several ways:

- The microorganisms might be contained in bodily

substances: semen, vaginal secretions, blood, saliva, urine, or feces.

- They might be present in discharges—cellular debris, pus, and white blood cells—from infectious sores.
- Or they might be transferred from infected skin like an ulcer (a crater in the skin).

Not infrequently, a disease might enter your body by more than one of these avenues. In any event, they make their way in through tiny scrapes or cuts in the skin that are always present, whether you can see them or not, or they might simply enter the urethra, the opening at the head of the penis.

We describe sores from STDs as being *vesicles* (small blisters that contain clear fluid), *pustules* (pimples that contain pus), or *ulcers* (open craters that might have discharges or be dry).

The significance of the method of infection becomes obvious when you think about symptoms. For a disease passed only from sores—as is the case with syphilis, for example—inspection of a person's genitals might reveal the risk. But a disease passed by bodily fluids—HIV, for example—will offer no warning signs. What's more, the transmission method determines whether a carrier is infectious only during outbreaks or at any time.

Because a number of STDs can be passed on by people who show no symptoms and who, in fact, might not even know they have the disease, "carriers" play an important role in their spread. Although it varies from disease to disease, in some cases as many as 70 percent of all people carrying a particular disease might be asymptomatic (a live wire) but infectious.

Blood transfusions, for example, can infect an otherwise low-risk person. The odds aren't high, but it can and does happen. That's why I advise my surgery patients to bank their own blood in advance if at all possible.

Who's at Risk?

I'm tempted to say that *everyone* is at risk of catching a sexually transmitted disease—even those who don't have sex. Blood transfusions, for example, can infect an otherwise low-risk person. The odds aren't high, but it can and does happen. That's why I advise my surgery patients to bank their own blood in advance if at all possible. Ask your physician how to do this if you're planning surgery.

Realistically, though, some people are at much greater risk than others. Among sexually active people, those who've been in a monogamous relationship for at least six months are at the lowest risk. As long as they take precautions for the first six months, are tested disease-free at the end of that waiting period, and remain exclusively monogamous, it's as safe a relationship as is practical. However, there is no guarantee attached to that six-month figure. HIV, for example, has at least six months' latency, but other STDs—genital warts, for one—might take years to appear.

I can't overemphasize the tragic results that can follow when a sexual disease invades a family. I've seen men happily married for years or even decades who swear to me that they and their wives have always been faithful. Then a wife turns up with an abnormal Pap smear indicating condyloma and pre-cancerous changes. I can only assume the condition goes back to their college days. Needless to say, such a discovery can destroy trust and faith, and damage a marriage. I've been asked to talk to divorce attorneys about my diagnosis of STD, and I've even testified in divorce cases that stemmed from an STD. It's a terrible way for a marriage to end.

Teach Your Children Well

As teenage pregnancies have increased and AIDS has threatened the population, we've seen a vigorous national debate on the best way of protecting our children. Is it abstinence or education? Do we simply tell them not to do it, or do we tell them how their bodies work and what can go wrong?

I know I'm going to ruffle a few feathers by saying so, but advocating abstinence alone isn't enough. Numerous reports tell us that more kids than ever before are having sex, and they're doing it younger than ever before. For every sexually transmitted disease, the most rapid growth in cases is among young people under twenty-five. Between 40 and 50 percent of our fifteen-year olds have had sex, yet only a third to half of them used condoms. Some experts estimate that as much as a quarter of all teenagers have one or another sexually transmitted disease. Add to that what so many parents already know about their own children, and you've got a problem that is not going to go away by just saying "No."

A study of ninth-graders in the Journal of Pediatr*ics* found that three factors predicted risky sexual behavior: 1) peer pressure, 2) alcohol and drug use, and 3) lack of knowledge about sexually transmitted diseases. We can and should try to influence our children to resist the first two factors, but we can only be sure of success with the third.

Yes, you should definitely tell your children that not having sex is the best way to avoid disease and unwanted pregnancy. But let's face facts: Many, many young people are having sex. They need to know how people get diseases and get pregnant, and how to avoid both. No sex is the only safe sex, but there is no excuse today for having unsafe sex.

Teaching your children how to protect themselves from sexually transmitted diseases isn't easy, but it's no more difficult than teaching them how to take care of themselves generally. Make it a part of general education about their bodies and their health. They'll be listening especially closely when you talk about the sexual parts, but you'll both be more at ease if sex is part of the discussion, not the whole thing.

Our point of view won't necessarily become our child's—especially if we try to dictate it. If you don't believe in premarital sex, say so. But you must arm your child with the knowledge to avoid the consequences if he or she disagrees and decides to have sex. They have to be responsible for their own actions—and when it comes to teenage boys, that's hard because they really live with that bulletproof mystique already discussed several times in this book. I know, because I have two boys, ages fourteen and sixteen. I trust them to drive cars and make other decisions. I try to give them the guidance and moral background, but the ultimate decision is theirs.

When you're talking to your kids about these vital matters, use the information found in the different steps of this book. Here are some pointers for discussing disease and sexuality:

The importance of diet (see Steps Four and Five for details)

When you talk about diet, you can mention that high-fat diets might lead to arterial disease, which leads to impotence. That opens the door to talking about how erections work and, therefore, how sex works.

The importance of exercise (again, review Steps Four and Five)

Exercise also can be tied to arterial disease, potency, and sex.

Self-examinations (see Step One)

When you talk about testicle and penis self-exams, bring up sexually transmitted diseases and what to look for; it opens the door to talking about how condoms protect from getting those diseases and also how they prevent pregnancy.

Understanding how family history affects risks to your health (see Step One)

Diabetes, for example, raises risk of potency problems; testicular cancer runs in families and increases the need for rigorous self-exams.

Ejaculation (see Step Six).

We discuss how erections and ejaculation occur, and how a contaminated body fluid can be passed from one person to another.

Truth—Or Consequences: Life After the Sexual Revolution

People who haven't entered into a monogamous relationship have a decision to make. Speaking as a doctor—no value judgments—I will tell you that abstinence is the only sure way to protect yourself from catching something through sex. You have to decide whether you want that ultimate protection. If you've chosen abstinence, some of the rest of this section will be irrelevant to you. If you decide to go ahead with sex, however, I have some strong suggestions.

First, let's get one thing straight: The sexual revolution is over. There's no place for spontaneous—let alone "free"—sex in the 1990s. At the very least, you should be doing the following any time you even consider having sex with a partner you've known less than six months:

1

Talk first about each other's sexual past.

You want assurance that your potential partner is disease-free, and you're perfectly within your rights to ask for evidence of negative tests. Bear in mind, however, that tests aren't foolproof. You also want to know that your prospective bedmate hasn't practiced risky behaviors. What are those?

- **Unprotected sex.**

- **Numerous partners. Women who have had more than twenty partners are 2.6 times as likely to have contracted herpes.**

- **Excessive alcohol consumption. A Bay Area study found that problem drinkers were almost four-and-a-half times more likely than moderate drinkers to get AIDS.**

- **Oral contraceptives. Women who use birth-control pills for longer than six months are at 2.4 times greater risk of getting chlamydia, independent of other risk factors.**

- **Anal intercourse. Because the anus is easily damaged during anal intercourse, the likelihood of disease transmission goes up.**

- Intravenous drug use. Independent of the risk of infection from shared needles, IV drug users are more likely to have a sexually transmitted disease.

- Having had a sexually transmitted disease, even if it's cured. One disease opens the doors for others, which might not have been treated.

2
Always use a condom and use it correctly.

Only latex or polyurethane non-novelty condoms protect against disease. Never use natural or exotic condoms for that purpose. Condoms lubricated with the spermicide nonoxynol-9 might increase protection against some diseases.

- Put the condom on before you have any contact with another person that involves the penis.

- Leave a space at the tip of the condom for semen and roll it all the way to the base of your penis.

- Never use an oil-based lubricant such as petroleum jelly, mineral or vegetable oil, or cold cream. That can break down the latex in the condoms.

- Withdraw your penis immediately after ejaculating (while it's still erect), holding the condom in place at the base of your penis.

- Never reuse a condom.

3
Suggest that your partner use barrier contraceptives.

Although neither of you thinks you have a disease, you might simply not be showing symptoms. Women who use a diaphragm or sponge increase their degree of protection from gonorrhea, chlamydia, and trichomoniasis over the use of a condom alone. Also consider using female condoms, which have been introduced recently.

4
Opt for less-risky sexual practices.

Oral sex (with protection in the form of a condom and dental dam) is less risky than vaginal intercourse, which is less risky than anal intercourse.

5

Be especially diligent about examining your genitals for sores or other irregularities (see Step One for a detailed description).

And see your doctor if you even suspect something's not quite right.

All about Condoms

During production, a random selection of condoms is subjected to several quality-control checks. Some are inflated with twenty-five liters of air, a common standard used to judge condoms in the U.S. and other countries. Others might be stretched lengthwise to test for breakage, and still others might be expanded in diameter by many times. A few might even be subjected to simulated intercourse on a machine designed to replicate a penis thrusting in a vagina.

A few might even be subjected to simulated intercourse on a machine designed to replicate a penis thrusting in a vagina.

With all that quality assurance, condom failures are rare. We know that condoms are about 98 percent effective for careful, experienced users, and at least 85 percent for the population as a whole. Most experts also agree that when a condom does fail, it's usually because it was too old or improperly stored.

Depending on how they're stored, latex condoms have a shelf life of between one and five years. Kept in the refrigerator, where it's cool and dry, they'll easily go full term. But in the tropics, without refrigeration, a year is the outside limit. Likewise, your wallet or the glove compartment of the car is no place to store a condom. Condoms have an expiration date stamped on their outer package—it might be for the condoms themselves or for the spermicide—but not usually on the individual foil packs, so it's important to hang onto that original box.

If you ever have any doubt about a condom's age or how it's been stored, don't depend on it!

Shopping Choices

Display racks give the impression that there's a bewildering array of choices to make when buying condoms. True, there are novelty condoms—textures, colors, even scents—but there are really only five functional options to consider: lubrication, spermicide, reservoir tip, thickness, and size.

Lubrication

Latex condoms are packaged dry or coated with a water-based silicone lubricant. This is purely a matter of personal preference, though if you choose to apply your own lubricant, it must not be petroleum based.

Spermicide

Nonoxynol-9, a chemical that kills sperm is now an option from most condom manufacturers. The spermicide offers some protection if semen leaks out into the vagina, though it's probably less effective than spermicidal foams placed in the vagina. In some cases, the spermicide serves as the lubricant; in others, a silicone lubricant is added. Besides boosting the effectiveness of a condom as a birth-control method, spermicide help protect against some STDs—especially HIV and hepatitis.

Reservoir Tip

Most condoms have a protrusion at the tip to leave room for semen when you ejaculate. You can achieve the same effect by leaving some slack when you don a nonreservoir condom, but the reservoir-tip models cost no more, so why not?

Thickness

Some condoms advertise that they're especially thin for increased sensitivity. Whatever the merits of this claim, decreasing the thickness of the latex will make the condom a little less durable. Likewise, condoms are available that are thicker than standard. You'll have to judge whether your sexual activities are sedate enough for thin condoms or energetic enough to merit added protection, although anal intercourse is certainly one practice that calls for a heavier-duty condom.

Size

It's not exactly like buying shoes yet, but manufacturers are beginning to offer condoms for men with larger-than-average penises. Mentor, for example, has the Magnum, which is maybe an eighth of an inch larger in diameter and three-quarters of an inch longer than the industry-standard 1 3/8-inch by 7 1/2-inch rubber. Most penises are about the same size when erect—six inches long on average—but larger men might find the new condoms more comfortable. (Remember, buying the bigger size might be good for your ego, but it must fit snugly enough to stay on.)

Alternative Condoms

So-called "natural" or "skin" condoms are made from a portion of a lamb's large intestine, called the cecum. Their claim to fame is increased sensitivity, an attribute that hasn't been confirmed in any sort of clinical trial. In any event, they are considerably more expensive than latex condoms and might not protect as effectively against some sexually transmitted diseases, such as AIDS and hepatitis B. In my opinion, the only compelling reason to use a natural condom rather than a latex one is if you or your partner is allergic to latex. (Perhaps as much as 5 percent of the population has some reaction to proteins in latex rubber. If you or your partner itch after sex or develop a rash, talk to your doctor.)

Female condoms are a recent development. The first one, the Reality Vaginal Pouch, was approved in 1992 by the Food and Drug Administration. Made from polyurethane rather than latex, the woman's version of the rubber goes inside the vagina. A ring positions the inner end around the cervix, and another ring on the outside keeps it in place. Testing shows them to be as effective at preventing pregnancy as latex condoms, but there is some evidence that they're not as good for disease prevention. Female condoms are more expensive than garden-variety latex, but they offer another alternative for people with latex allergies.

A Few Words—and Some Numbers—In Favor of Abstinence.

I hope by now I've convinced those of you who are sexually active and not monogamous for at least six months that your risk of catching something is very real. And I hope you're saying, "You bet I'm going to use a condom." But I'm afraid I'm going to have to burst even that bubble of hope. Herpes and genital warts, for example, are very sneaky diseases. You can catch either by contacting parts of the body that won't be protected by a condom—the area around the base of the penis, the buttocks, or in between. A study of couples where one person had herpes found that 10 percent of the partners became infected within a year, despite *always* using condoms and abstaining when the herpes was active. As the following chart shows, that's a lot better than no protection, but it proves that the only truly safe sex is no sex—and as I said earlier, there's no excuse for unsafe sex.

RISK OF INFECTION (%) FROM ONE UNPROTECTED ENCOUNTER		
	Men	Women
Genital Herpes	30	30
Gonorrhea	25	50
Chlamydia	20	40
Syphilis	20	30
Chancroid	15	30
Genital Warts	10	10
Hepatitis B	5	10
HIV	0.9	1

Source: Health and Sexuality

A Brief Rogue's Gallery

I f you suspect you've been infected, it's very important that you be thoroughly tested to determine which disease you might have, since treatment must be tailored to the disease. That's why

I've also mentioned what sort of test is used to diagnose each disease. Most are detected by direct inspection of material under a microscope, a blood test that looks for antigens (evidence that your body was trying to fight something), or a culture (growing more of the organism in an enhanced environment until it becomes easier to see).

If you suspect you've been infected, it's very important that you be thoroughly tested to determine which disease you might have, since treatment must be tailored to the disease.

At the same time, you need to understand the limitations of testing. There is no such thing as a "standard panel" to cover all the diseases. To do every test possible would be frightfully expensive, and it still wouldn't absolutely prove that you have or don't have a disease. We can test for herpes, for example, by looking for antigens in your blood. But the presence of antigens proves only that you might have had one of the herpes viruses in your system at one time. It could have been a cold sore.

What can a careless fling get you? I see the results thirty or forty times a month at the Male Health Center. I've diagnosed STDs in boys as young as fifteen and men well into their seventies. The following collection *(see page 208)* of bacterial, viral, fungal, and other infections, along with an insect infestation, are just the most common sexually transmitted diseases.

ESTIMATED INCIDENCE AND PREVALENCE OF SELECTED SEXUALLY TRANSMITTED DISEASES (STDS) IN 1992		
STD	Incidence (per year)	Prevalence (total)
Gonorrhea (GC)	1,100,000	Not available
Syphilis	120,000	Not available
Congenital Syphilis	3,500	Not available
Chlamydia (CT)	4,000,000	Not available
Human Papillomavirus (Condyloma)	500,000 - 1,000,000	At least 24,000,000
Genital Herpes	200,000 - 500,000	At least 31,000,000
Trichomoniasis	3,000,000	Not available
Hepatitis B	100,000 - 200,000	Not available
Urethritis (non-GC, non-CT)	1,200,000	Not available
Mucopurulent cervicitis (non-GC, non-CT)	1,000,000	Not available
Reported AIDS cases*	45,472	140,000 - 168,000**
HIV infection	Not available	1,000,000

* Based on cases reported through September 1992

* Number of persons diagnosed with AIDS who were still alive at some time in 1992

(Source: The Centers for Disease Control and Prevention)

AIDS

The human immunodeficiency virus (HIV) breaks down the body's defenses against many diseases, producing a condition called acquired immune deficiency syndrome, or AIDS. HIV infection is not obvious in laboratory tests for up to six months, and AIDS symptoms might take years to develop.

How Contracted About three-quarters of all AIDS cases are acquired sexually. Heterosexual infection is the fastest-growing category. An HIV carrier often has no symptoms.

Effects Thus far, HIV infection appears always to lead eventually to AIDS, which is always fatal.

Diagnosis Blood tests (two).

Treatment There is no cure, but several drugs might prolong life and reduce suffering. There are rapid developments in this area.

Candidiasis (yeast infection)	A fungal infection that a man—only rarely a circumcised man—might harbor and pass back to his female partner. Symptoms in men are usually minor (maybe a rash), unless the man has diabetes or an immune system problem, but candidiasis accounts for 90 percent of vaginal infections.
How Contracted	Fungi are directly transferred between genitals.
Effects	Minor or nonexistent in most men. Most also turn out to be free of fungi when sent to me for testing.
Diagnosis	Examination of scrapings under microscope or culture.
Treatment	Over-the-counter fungal preparations. Use a condom if you suspect you're reinfecting your partner.

Chancroid	A bacterial infection that develops four to fourteen days after exposure and resembles syphilis in early stages. Chancroid, however, rapidly becomes infected, has an irregular border, and is usually painful.
How Contracted	Contagious only when sores are active.
Frequency	Less common than syphilis in the U.S., but very common in tropical countries. U.S. incidence increased nearly tenfold between 1984 and 1987.
Effects	Can produce whole-body symptoms, including fever and swollen lymph nodes.
Diagnosis	Microscopic examination of scrapings, followed by culture.
Treatment	Erythromycin or ceftriaxone.

Chlamydia	A newcomer, chlamydia bacterial infection is now the most commonly reported sexually transmitted disease, with over four million new cases each year. About a quarter of men and three-quarters of women never develop symptoms. Those who do experience burning on urination, a clear-to-creamy dis-

	charge from the tip of the penis, and sometimes itching seven to twenty-eight days after exposure.
How Contracted	Infectious at any time, even when no symptoms appear.
Effects	Numerous problems in pregnant women. Sterility in men and women. Urethral, prostate, and epididymal problems in men.
Diagnosis	Most commonly cell culture or blood test.
Treatment	Tetracycline, erythromycin, or quinolones.

Condyloma	A type of viral wart that occurs on the genitals, some forms of condyloma produce visible warts. Others (the most dangerous types) might be invisible to the naked eye. Warts, if there are any to be seen, don't show up for one to three months (or a lot longer) after exposure. They might be much more common than previously thought; one test of college women showed that almost half had condyloma.
How Contracted	Human pappilomaviruses are so prevalent because of their very efficient transmission—up to about a ten-percent chance in one encounter. Symptoms need not be present.
Effects	Some types of condyloma have been strongly associated with cervical cancer in women and penile cancer in men.
Diagnosis	Often found through a woman's Pap smear; otherwise only through visual inspection with enhancement. We can also wrap the penis in a cloth saturated with a mild vinegar or acid solution, wait five minutes, and look with a microscope. The condyloma can stain white.
Treatment	There is no cure, but warts might be removed with caustic solutions, creams, freezing, burning, lasers, or surgery, which might reduce cancer risk.

Genital Herpes	Groups of painful small bumps break out on the head, shaft, and base of penis, usually within twelve days (but sometimes much longer) of exposure to this virus. Other sites in the genital area or on the mouth might develop sores. There are two types: I and II. About 90 percent of genital herpes are Type II, the more dangerous variety.
How Contracted	Most contagious when sores are present, but it might be passed from one person to another when no symptoms are present.
Effects	Outbreaks might recur unpredictably, but usually five to eight times per year, causing painful sores and whole-body flulike symptoms. Herpes can be fatal to the newborn.
Diagnosis	Microscopic examination of scrapings or a blood test.
Treatment	There is no cure, but acyclovir reduces symptoms and will lessen recurrences if taken regularly.
Gonorrhea	A bacterial infection that develops in one to ten days. There might be no symptoms at all—especially in women—or there might be burning on urination and a clear-to-cloudy discharge from the tip of the penis.
How Contracted	Infectious at any time, even when there are no symptoms.
Effects	If not treated promptly, it might invade other parts of the urinary tract. Narrowing of the urethra or sterility might result.
Diagnosis	Culture.
Treatment	Single dose of ceftriaxone, spectinomycin, or quinolones, followed by week-long treatment with doxycycline, tetracycline, or erythromycin.

Hepatitis	About a quarter of all hepatitis-B viral infections come from sexual contact, producing tiredness, muscle and joint pain, sore throat, fever, and gastrointestinal distress six weeks to six months after exposure.
How Contracted	Infectious at any time, including before the onset of first symptoms. Might be transmitted on saliva, semen, feces, or urine.
Effects	Causes liver inflammation, which can lead to loss of function or liver cancer.
Diagnosis	Blood test.
Treatment	A newly approved drug, interferon alpha-2b, seems to help many people with hepatitis-B. Those who might have been exposed should receive immune serum globulin to reduce outbreaks.
Pubic Lice	Crab lice are small insects that take up residence in pubic hair—and occasionally in hair on the head, beard, buttocks, thighs, or eyebrows. They produce itching and a rash about a month after exposure.
How Contracted	Crab lice cross from one person to another during sexual contact.
Effects	Usually minor, although there can be infections.
Diagnosis	Visual inspections.
Treatment	Over-the-counter preparations of the natural insecticide pyrethrin or prescription lindane.

Syphilis	An infection that starts as a painless ulcer, which then disappears, and subsequently comes back as a dull red rash on the body about six months after the first episode. Once the rash disappears, internal organs might become infected and begin to deteriorate.
How Contracted	Contagious only when sores are active.
Effects	Can be fatal if not treated promptly.
Diagnosis	Blood test.
Treatment	Penicillin, tetracycline, or erythromycin.

Trichomoniasis	An infection by a protozoan (single-celled animal), trichomoniasis infects about 70 percent of all men who have sex with an infected woman, but most men get rid of the infection naturally within a few weeks. Women develop a foul-smelling vaginal discharge, but symptoms—pain on urination and discharge—develop in only 5 to 10 percent of men.
How Contracted	Contagious at any time, even when there are no symptoms.
Effects	Infertility and irritation.
Diagnosis	Microscopic exam of discharge; sometimes a culture.
Treatment	Metronidazole is usually very effective.

Ureaplasma Urealyticum	Similar to chlamydia in symptoms and development, ureaplasma has also only been recognized in recent years as a disease distinct from gonorrhea. The discharge from ureaplasma might have a more distinctive whitish appearance, and women might develop lower abdominal pain. Women rarely have symptoms, however, while they are somewhat more frequent in men. About 80 percent of women and 34 percent of men might carry it without knowing.
How Contracted	Infectious at any time, even when there are no symptoms.

Effects	Sterility, miscarriage, and premature birth in women. Prostate problems in men. Might also be involved in rheumatic diseases, such as infectious arthritis.
Diagnosis	Difficult; must be carefully cultured. Rule out others first.
Treatment	Doxycycline or quinolones.

Nonspecific Urethritis	A catchall classification for the roughly 10 percent of urinary infections for which we can't find a cause.
How Contracted	Might be sexual, but we're not sure.
Effects	Irritation.
Diagnosis	Process of elimination.
Treatment	Most respond to antibiotics.

Taking Responsibility

Getting a sexually transmitted disease gives you more than disease and heartbreak; it gives you *responsibility.* You really must let every partner you've had know that they might have been exposed. How far you go back depends on the particular disease and when *you* might have been exposed. Some STDs can remain dormant in your body for years before causing symptoms, during which time you can infect others.

Talk to your doctor about it, and ask for advice about how to relay the news. You're not alone. Your doctor is your health ally, and he or she is also responsible for helping you see that the disease goes no further. At the same time, be aware that you and your health partner might be learning to cope with your sexually transmitted disease together. Most doctors have not been trained in the person-to-person management of this problem, so you might have to encourage him or her to give you all the facts

Contacting partners— present and past—will not be fun, but it's the most caring thing you can do. And even if you're now in a monogamous relationship, it's the only way you can avoid passing the disease back and forth between the two of you—the "ping-pong" effect.

about your condition. It's worth working on that dialogue, though, because knowledge will give you power. And if your doctor just isn't helpful on this very sensitive subject . . . well, that's what the Yellow Pages are for. Remember that "question authority" attitude we discussed in Step Two? If you are not able to communicate, if you feel he or she is not taking you seriously, if you aren't getting answers— it's time to seek help elsewhere.

Be sure to ask about support groups, because you are far from alone. There are national organizations that sponsor local groups for both herpes and genital warts. There is a national herpes hot line and a national STD hotline. At the end of this step, I'll give you several numbers to call.

Contacting partners—present and past—will not be fun, but it's the most caring thing you can do. And even if you're now in a monogamous relationship, it's the only way you can avoid passing the disease back and forth between the two of you—the "ping-pong" effect.

With your current partner(s), a proper approach can help. Pick a private, quiet moment when there's plenty of time for discussion. Don't point fingers. Accusing your partner of giving you the disease won't help. Instead, say something like, "I found some bumps on my penis and went to the doctor to be tested. The doctor says I have herpes. It's not life-threatening, but it's very serious, and—you need to be checked too."

Be specific about which STD it is. Stress that early detection reduces later hazards, and explain what testing involves. Be positive, and emphasize that you want to work the problem out together.

By the time you're relaying these messages to past partners, you'll be an expert. So remember how afraid you were when you first came in for testing. Fear of the unknown is much worse than the reality. By passing on what you've learned, you can help ease the way for others.

Q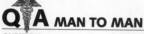A MAN TO MAN

QUESTION	ANSWER
Is it possible to get the clap from a toilet seat?	It's within the realm of possibility, but it's about as likely as winning the state lottery. The bacterium Neisseria gonorrhea can only survive outside the friendly domain of the urinary tract or vagina for about an hour. Add to that the complication of getting the bacteria from the toilet seat into your genitals, and the odds go even lower. I suspect that nonsexual transmission of the clap only happens in the minds of men who desperately want some explanation for what they've got.

QUESTION	ANSWER
If I have burning on urination, should I automatically go to the doctor?	If that burning sensation lasts more than a day, or if you have any risk factors for a sexually transmitted disease—anything other than completely monogamous sexual relations for at least three years—definitely. Men so infrequently acquire benign urinary tract infections that resolve without treatment, that you'd be better off going in to have your doctor check out the possibilities. Women, on the other hand, sometimes have some genital irritation that doesn't require anything more than adequate fluids to correct.

QUESTION	ANSWER
Since some of the strains of human papillomavirus pose more risk than others, isn't it important to know which one(s) you have?	Ideally, we would like to know which HPV types you have, but practically we can't. We tell the various HPV apart according to their genetic code (DNA), and it takes a sophisticated and very expensive—hundreds of dollars—test called polymerase chain reaction (PCR) to reveal DNA. At that, PCR sometimes misses the mark, which might unduly cause alarm if a dangerous strain turned up. Until we have an economical, practical test for typing, we'll have to depend on prevention and the limited treatments we have.

QUESTION	ANSWER
I have heard that some urethral infections can cause male infertility. Is there anything to this?	Chlamydia's (and ureaplasma's) association with pelvic inflammatory disease and subsequent sterility is backed by pretty strong evidence. In men, however, the data are much less conclusive. Russian doctors have found ureaplasma in about a third of men and women seeking help with fertility problems. And they note abnormalities in the sperm that disappear after antibiotic treatment. And a study of couples visiting an in-vitro-fertilization clinic has shown that couples in which either the man or the woman has ureaplasma are less likely to conceive. Frankly, I think the jury's still out. We just haven't studied ureaplasma enough to know clearly what all its effects might be. One thing we are sure of, though, is that chlamydia can cause urethral strictures—deformities in or narrowing of the male urethra—which can be serious problems requiring surgical correction.

QUESTION	ANSWER
Even the best-fitting condoms reduce the physical pleasure of sexual intercourse. Is there any way around that while still fulfilling my male share of the load in taking precautions against sexually transmitted diseases?	Condom manufacturers are experimenting with new thinner, more sensitive condoms, and although they are not yet available, it is anticipated that they will be released in the near future. The only other option, unfortunately, is the female condom, which according to my patients is not associated with any increased sensitivity for the man. At this time, there really is no way around the condom issue, but once again remember it is important to use latex, not animal skin.

QUESTION	ANSWER
What are the dangers of masturbation in terms of disease, if any?	To my knowledge, there is no danger with masturbation in general. However, excessive masturbation—and I have seen patients who masturbate three or four times a day—is not normal and frequently is associated with abnormal social behavior. Also, masturbation to the exclusion of developing personal relationshipsis obviously not necessarily in one's best interests. While there is nothing sinful or evil about masturbation, it's obviously a very solitary, introverted act. The best sex, as we've discussed, comes in mutually supportive relationships. Additionally, there are rare cases of individuals using abnormal force in order to masturbate. I have seen cases where the penis has been injured in these situations.

QUESTION	ANSWER
Can sexually transmitted diseases be transmitted mouth to mouth in something as simple as a kiss?	If the sexually transmitted disease is present in the secretions, transmission—in theory—through saliva, not contact with the lips, is possible. I have seen and treated men who have developed warts of condyloma in their mouths.

QUESTION	ANSWER
I've heard all kinds of things regarding the "waiting period" between exposure to HIV and the appearance of AIDS-related symptoms. Some experts say six months; others say it could take up to ten years. What's the real deal?	There is no single waiting period or safety period. It can take at least six months for an HIV test to become positive after exposure. On the other hand, individuals who have been exposed can go years before their tests become positive. While certainly no news is good news, it does not assure us that there is no problem.

HOTLINES	
AIDS Hotline	• **(800) 243-2437**
Center for Disease Control	• **(404) 639-3311**
Herpes Hotline	• **(919) 361-8488**
HPV (Condyloma) Support Program	• **(919) 361-8400**
Sexually Transmitted Disease Hotline	• **(800) 227-8922**

8

Relating to Family, Friends, and Fellow Man

CONCLUSION: NO MAN IS AN ISLAND

WOMEN TALK: Ruth Jenkins, age fifty-seven

Wally had had a potency problem for five years or so. Being a nurse, I knew enough to understand that these things usually have some physical basis, but it still hurt a lot. He started avoiding any sort of closeness. He wouldn't cuddle, and he'd go to bed early. I think it's natural for any woman to assume that if her man can't get an erection, he doesn't find her attractive any more. And when he stops paying any attention at all, well, you figure he's not interested in you as a person either. I tried to get him to go to a doctor, but he'd just huff and refuse.

"It took a really serious problem to finally get his attention. I knew something was wrong on Saturday, but he even denied it when I asked him. 'Nope, I'm okay,' he'd say. It's this 'I'm bulletproof' attitude he's got: 'I'm a man; I'm not supposed to get sick.' And I think it's especially bad when it's a male problem.

"So he sat there most of the weekend hardly able to move and not eating a thing. Do you know how terrible it made me feel seeing him hurt that much? It wasn't until the middle of the night Sunday that it finally got so bad that he admitted he was having trouble.

"It turned out he hadn't been able to urinate since Saturday morning. I packed him into the car and got him to the emergency room where they took care of the acute retention problem. His prostate was so *enlarged, though, that the doctor thought an operation was necessary—a transurethral resection, what a lot of men call a roto-rooter job. I thought he'd completely fall apart when the doctor told him he had to have surgery, but he got through it.*

"In a way, the prostate problem has turned out to be a blessing. He liked the doctor a lot, and after the surgery he even talked to him about his erection difficulties. The doctor has been helping him out with that, and it's done wonders for his attitude to be having erections again. I can't complain either, but the best part for me has been the improvement in his attitude about life. We're friends again. He tells me about what happens to him at work, and we share some laughs about the situations that come up in my nursing work. We enjoy being together, sitting next to each other, because there's no longer that pressure on him. He's not worried that a situation will develop where he'll fail to perform.

"Another thing we've started doing is getting together with some other people who've had similar experiences, and Wally's even started talking about what he went through—how lonely he felt, how he thought if he ignored his problems they might go away. It's pretty amazing to see him telling other guys that they can get through their troubles. They're not alone."

What's a woman's commentary doing in a book about male health? The fact is, guys, we're in this together. That means you and me, and it also means the women and children who share our lives. Really, it's a two-way street: What we do with our health affects them, and the way we get along with them has powerful, although subtle effects on our health.

The other seven parts of this book describe steps you can take—things you can do that will lead to a longer, healthier, more satisfying life. In this last chapter, we need to take what we've learned and talk about putting it to work.

> *In a very real sense, it's not just changes in medicine that make it possible for men to live longer and better; it's changes in men.*

By now, you know that living longer is not that difficult to do. So, why in the world didn't someone write this book twenty or thirty years ago? The answer, of course, is that no one would have listened. The time was not right. In a very real sense, it's not just changes in *medicine* that make it possible for men to live longer and better; it's changes in men.

Gradually, as women have begun to redefine their roles in society and the household, we have begun to redefine ours. Warren Farrell, in his controversial book, *The Myth of Male Power*, points out that the man's role is no longer exclusively to defend and provide for the people (women) who raise the children, thus ensuring our genetic future. Men are beginning to share the roles of nurturing and nesting, just as women are beginning to share the roles of soldier and breadwinner.

For the first time in human history (at least the recorded portion), men aren't called on to be what Farrell calls the disposable sex. We are not expected to give our lives—whether it be in battle or working at a grueling, dangerous job—for our families. Admittedly, we've only made a start. We have a very long way to go. But the door is open for us to redefine what it is to be a man.

This book isn't the place to discuss the men's movement, although I believe that its basic themes—that men have rights, too, and that we need to talk to each other about what we feel—are very important. Thankfully, our goals here are much simpler. We just need to identify some of the Dark Ages attitudes and ways of behaving that hold us back from living longer and getting along better with our partners, our children and our fellow men. It's time for us to replace those Dark Ages attitudes with space-age attitudes and ways of behaving.

First, let's consider what is really important to us. Do our greatest joys come from our jobs, our tidy yards, our golf handicaps, the fish we catch, or even our children's grade-point averages? I don't think so.

I believe they come from the human interactions we have with people while we work, play, and raise children. Without others to share our achievements, they're hollow and unsatisfying.

The same thing goes for your health. Excellent fitness and long life won't mean much without the joy of sharing it with others. And that sharing means that your health is not yours alone to throw away.

If you have casual sex, it's not just you who might get a sexually transmitted disease. Your partner could end up with an incurable disease or cervical cancer as a result of your indiscretion. If you smoke cigarettes, subsist on potato chips and beer, and exercise nothing more than your index finger on the remote control, it won't just ruin your health. When you become impotent because your arteries clog up, chances are your partner will feel as much pain and loss as you do. And if you die young from all these bad habits, you will not only create a widow. Perhaps even worse, you also will have taught your children how to follow in your footsteps. It's a legacy you don't want to leave.

If that sounds like a heavy responsibility, try instead to think of it as a terrific opportunity. Health is like love in this way: When you share it with someone else, you don't have less, you have more—and better. And unlike a contract that's done when it's signed, or a fish that's caught and cooked, or a perfect putt at the eighteenth hole, this job is never finished, because this job is life itself. All you have to do is try. Take care of yourself and work on taking care of the significant others in your life: your partner, your children, and your fellow man.

Excellent fitness and long life won't mean much without the joy of sharing it with others. And that sharing means that your health is not yours alone to throw away.

Your Relationship, and Sex

Nature gave us the pleasure of sex to enjoy, and at the risk of overemphasizing it, I think it's a terrible shame when people go without sex for no good reason. Sex is an integral part of the "better" I'm talking about when I say you can "live longer and live better."

During the week I was finishing this book, I saw two men in their mid-thirties who had no sex lives. One had not been able to function in more than ten years, and he was living like a hermit. The other had *never* had sexual intercourse. Both men were, with help, fully capable of having satisfying sexual relationships. Without erections, both men felt like they were among the walking dead. Now they've awakened.

An erection, of course, is the starting point for sex. But truly good sex—the kind that is more than just biological function—can happen only within the atmosphere of a good relationship. What is the fundamental difference between sex and good sex? Simple. Emotion. Sex without feelings—without a caring interaction with your partner—is simply the reproductive urge in action. It lasts only a few minutes, offers no long-term satisfaction, and makes small use of the opportunities we're given to enjoy more.

Good sex and good relationships might be inseparable, but that doesn't mean they happen naturally. Sex is an instinct, but good sex (and good relationships) must be learned and practiced. When we have a good relationship, we can have good sex, which increases the bond between man and woman. It helps us form a cooperative partnership that benefits both individuals and provides children with an environment where they're more likely to thrive. Good relationships and good sex exist because they make us happy and increase the odds of us and our genes surviving.

One reason that good sex and good relationships don't come without effort is that men and women have tended to see them as occurring in different order. Both men and women are interested in sex, but their approaches to it are different.

It's sort of a chicken-or-the-egg question: Men get close through sex, while women express the closeness they feel through sex. In general, women are much less focused on sex; they're focused on relationships, face-to-face sharing of cares, concerns, and joys. When they feel connected with their partner and cared for, they can become highly aroused and have great sex. We men have been taught to be less patient. We work side by side to compete and achieve goals. In sex, we tend to want to get on with it. It's not easy for us to slow down, communicate, and enjoy the intimacy that precedes good sex.

> *In sex, we tend to want to get on with it. It's not easy for us to slow down, communicate, and enjoy the intimacy that precedes good sex.*

We also exist in a society that perpetuates illusions about what men are and should be. In his book *The New Male Sexuality,* Dr. Bernie Zilbergeld has identified a dozen myths about men and sex that pretty much summarize the major hurdles we face in improving our relationships.

DR. ZILBERGELD'S TWELVE MYTHS ABOUT SEX	
Myth Number 1	We're liberated and very comfortable about sex.
	FACT: On the contrary, most Americans are quite uncomfortable with open discussion of sex. Why else would we permit savage violence on television while censoring sex? Believing that we are liberated when we aren't leads to narrow-mindedness and inability to change.
Myth Number 2	A real man doesn't express his feelings.
	FACT: If you can't express your feelings, you can't have more than biological sex.
Myth Number 3	All touching is sexual.
	FACT: Nonsexual touching is a fundamental human need. It soothes us and makes us feel cared for. We recognize that small children need it. Why shouldn't adults?
Myth Number 4	A man is always interested in and ready for sex.
	FACT: Men are just people—people who get tired, have rough days, and get distracted. Allow yourself to be human.
Myth Number 5	A real man performs in sex.
	FACT: Too many men view sex as something that proves they're men—not as a way to express caring or even lust. Performance reduces sex to hardware and measurements, which isn't good sex.

Myth Number 6	Sex is centered on a hard penis and what is done with it.
	FACT: Many of us never get over the fixation on the penis that being an adolescent male demands. Don't forget the other 95 percent of your body—and especially your brain.
Myth Number 7	Sex equals intercourse.
	FACT: Good sex isn't just genital, it includes hands, eyes, and talking—all ways in which we can share pleasure.
Myth Number 8	A man should always be able to give his partner an orgasm.
	FACT: Women *have* orgasms; we don't *give* them orgasms. Being concerned about your partner's pleasure is important, but an orgasm is not the only measure of success.
Myth Number 9	Good sex requires that the man have an orgasm.
	FACT: Sex and ejaculation have always been accepted as synonymous. Why? An automatic response of the nervous system is not by itself good sex.
Myth Number 10	Men don't have to listen to women during sex.
	FACT: Consider the possibility that a woman might mean what she says. She might not want to; she might not care if she didn't have an orgasm. She is a person.
Myth Number 11	Good sex is spontaneous and nonverbal.
	FACT: Only in Hollywood. Planning sex can add anticipation—not to mention increasing the likelihood that it will actually happen. And talk during sex can be a real stimulant. You are not attending a funeral.
Myth Number 12	Real men don't have sexual problems.
	FACT: Many men assume that admitting to a problem makes them less masculine and less desirable. Often times, the opposite is the case. Admitting to a problem humanizes a man. It's high time real men were allowed to be human.

This is not a quiz, but ask yourself how many of these myths you believe. One? Five? All twelve? Don't be ashamed to admit it; these myths are created by the very real sexual pressures we men feel. Women's liberation is essential and long overdue, but at the same time, the blame cast on men has had many negative effects on us—and

Through words, you must let her know that you are there to support her, that you value her mind as well as her body, that she is your best friend. You tell your friend how you feel, and you listen when she tells you how she feels. Honesty is what matters.

on our relationships. For example, women do deserve sexual pleasure as much as men, but too many men have felt a heavy obligation to deliver it. The myths of performance have been the result. We need to put these myths aside so we can attend to our relationships.

In a word, good relationships are about communication. Bringing home a paycheck and getting an erection are not enough. Through words, you must let her know that you are there to support her, that you value her mind as well as her body, that she is your best friend. You tell your friend how you feel, and you listen when she tells you how she feels. Honesty is what matters. Share your concerns with her, and let her know clearly when she has pleased you. If she hurts you, don't sulk. Tell her, but do it in unaccusing ways. You don't always have to agree, but you do need to avoid the sort of warfare that consists of attacking and defending.

I'm not just preaching here. Speaking as a doctor, I've seen many men reap the health benefits that flow from strong, supportive relationships. When these men, suffering from prostate cancer, impotence, or other male problems, come to the Male Health Center, their women come with them. They come together for the examinations and the pre-operative tests. They keep a vigil at the hospital during the surgery, and after the surgery is done, they come to the support group meetings and the post-operative visits. These men usually do very well—and I believe it's in part because of their strong, caring partners.

It's not easy being a man in a world where it's so unclear what a man is supposed to be, but the rewards of stepping beyond our traditional male roles are many. Not only do we live longer, but we get along better with those around us. And I can assure you, the better you get along with your partner, the better your sex life will be.

Your Children: Ensuring the Future

Although we are making great progress in re-defining who we are as men, we live with a tremendous amount of baggage from the years we've put in on this planet. Try as we might, we will never entirely shrug off the attitudes that our culture has given us. But with our children we have the opportunity to create a new norm. Think how much your father's actions influenced what you see as normal and correct. As fathers, we can set an example for our sons to follow, and we can create expectations in our daughters of what a man (and a husband) should be.

Each of us would probably come up with a slightly different image of what the ideal man should be, but I think we can agree on a few of the characteristics.:

- **He is loving and compassionate.**
- **He believes in himself.**
- **He is curious about the world around him.**
- **He enjoys life.**
- **He is a role model for the young.**
- **He takes care of himself (hopefully by following the steps in this book).**

Those are tall orders, but they're all attributes we would like our children to see in us and imitate.

In some cases, however, just setting a good example isn't enough. You need to educate your children, and you need to start at an early age. Who do you want to teach your children about sex? As former Surgeon General Dr. C. Everett Koop, said, "Proper teaching [about sex] is too important to be left to the schools. . . ." *You* need to teach your children to understand how their bodies work and to be proud of them.

This is a case where "just say no" doesn't get it. Sure, it's fine to promote abstinence, but it's far from adequate. Young people are having intercourse sooner and with more partners as each year passes. And for the first time in a decade, condom sales actually fell in 1991. While no sex might be the only truly safe sex, we must accept and deal with the reality. Listen to one of my teenage patients:

MEN TALK: Jerry Franks, age nineteen

really thought it wouldn't happen to me. You know, I tried always to use a condom, but I guess trying wasn't good enough.

"It was only one time, I think. I met this girl at a club and we went to her house. I used a condom, but later we wanted to do it again, and I didn't have another one. So we just did it. That was two months ago, and now I've got herpes.

"The doctor says there's no way to cure it. I knew there were diseases you could get—like AIDS or the clap—but I figured I wasn't very likely to get one. It's guys who have sex with prostitutes who get diseases. Well, and me, I guess.

"What's really going to be difficult is telling my current girlfriend. I met her only a couple of weeks after that one-night stand, and she's the first girl I've really felt like settling down with—at least for a while. I'm really scared that she might already have gotten herpes from me. But the doctor says I've got to tell her, and I know I do. She'll probably drop me. I guess I deserve it.

"I don't know how I'm going to get my life together after this. I can't imagine having sex with anybody. I think I'm growing up in a big hurry. Hey guys, take my word for it: It can happen to you and it only takes one mistake."

certainly don't want one of my sons to end up in that situation. Believe me, though, Jerry isn't unusual. I see boys regularly with herpes, condyloma, gonorrhea, and the host of other diseases that promiscuity can bring.

Why isn't the message about safe sex getting through? It's obvious: Our young people aren't convinced. They aren't fully educated about the risks, and they have a bulletproof mentality. Don't just tell them about AIDS, expecting that alone to persuade them. Statistics show that AIDS isn't a real threat in the minds of most young people.

Be sure your adolescents understand what you learned in Step Seven: AIDS is just one of several incurable sexually transmitted diseases. Make sure that your daughters know that two things independently increase their risk of developing female cancers—the age at which they begin having intercourse and the number of partners they have. And by all means, tell them that condoms are fine, but they're much less effective at protecting against some diseases than others.

Not until young people are taught how their bodies work and what the choices and risks really mean can they be expected to act sensibly. Parents need to educate and encourage their schools to educate.

Twenty years ago, saying "Don't do it because it's not nice" didn't work. Today, saying "Don't do it because you might get AIDS" isn't working. Instead, we need to say "Here are the facts; you decide." The more they know, the more abstinence will look like a real option.

At the same time, you owe your children more than scare tactics. Wouldn't it be wonderful if children grew up thinking that sex really is a great gift—one that is to be shared with the most important people in their lives? Let's face it, you won't convince them sex doesn't feel good. But if you can convey your own sense of wonder in it, and explain the difference between biology and sex in a stable, loving relationship, you'll have done the best anyone can to help them to decide to wait.

If you want to succeed, you won't lecture. You'll express your genuine concern for their well-being, and you'll let them know you understand how difficult the choices are and how heavy the pressure can be. Be your child's confidante, not his or her commander. Communication, understanding, and feeling are the messages you want to give and the traits you hope will rub off. Show them how it's done; there's nothing more instructive than a good example.

Your Fellow Man: Don't Beat Him; Join Him

For most of us, I think it's even more difficult to communicate honestly and sincerely with our fellow men than with our partners and children. When men do "guy things," it usually consists of an exchange of taunts, boasts, and shoulder punches. We've been taught that other men are our competitors—for our women, our jobs, and, in effect, even our masculinity. And we've been taught that we must be strong to survive. It starts all the way back in junior high locker rooms, continues at the lunch table, and carries right on through to the country club locker room and the health club at the YMCA. Men develop ways of dealing with each other that avoid real communication and establish a pecking order.

This book is as much about giving up those attitudes and actions as it is about taking control of your health. The two must go hand in hand. Exercise and healthful eating aren't going to save our skins unless we stop gritting our teeth and allow ourselves to feel. Medical science is beginning to show direct ways that our attitudes affect our health. You've probably heard of Type-A personalities—the aggressive, tense, competitive type—and the fact that such people seem more prone to having heart attacks. Now researchers have been able to record actual physiological effects that could lead the strong, silent-type man to get heart disease.

It's not easy to turn around ingrained behaviors, and the world can be a competitive, cutthroat place

Exercise and healthful eating aren't going to save our skins unless we stop gritting our teeth and allow ourselves to feel. Medical science is beginning to show direct ways that our attitudes affect our health.

at times. But there are also examples of men who have learned to relate to each other in new ways. One of them is a man I've had the good fortune to work with to help other men. Meet Ed Kaps, founder of Us Too, the prostate cancer support group.

MEN TALK: Ed Kaps

I was a successful automotive executive the first time I was told I had prostate cancer. At the time, I didn't let the impact of that sink in. After a course of radiation treatments, I got back to work and put the experience behind me. But ten years later the cancer was back, and this time I was told radiation wasn't going to be sufficient. In 1989 I entered a Chicago hospital to have a radical prostatectomy—my prostate, which lies between the bladder and the penis, was to be removed in surgery lasting several hours.

"Frankly, I was terrified. I'd just reached retirement age, and I'd managed to put away a tidy nest egg so I could enjoy my later years—quite a few of them, I had hoped. Lying in bed, I was convinced I was going to die. Because I was so scared, I talked to some of the hospital staff about what I was facing, and I realized how much it helped just to talk. We agreed that men facing a life-threatening situation really ought to have someone to talk to—that stewing in one's own worry wasn't helpful.

"My surgeon, Dr. Gerald Chodak, was impressed enough with what was developing in my hospital room that he decided to hold a get-together for men with prostate cancer. He sent letters to all his patients, and, much to our surprise, twenty-five men showed up for the first meeting in February of 1990. That turned out to be the first chapter of Us Too, a name we derived from Why Me?, the breast cancer support group.

"As it turns out, I never have gotten around to retiring. With my cofounder, Edward G. von Holst, I began answering more and more phone calls from doctors anxious to start prostate cancer support *groups in their areas. When Mr. von Holst died, on July 11, 1992, I took over completely and by the end of that year, more than one hundred Us Too offshoots had sprung up around the United States and foreign countries. Since then it's just been a steady forward march to bring Us Too's compassion to more and more men with prostate cancer.*

"What does Us Too do? Its number-one mission is for men with prostate cancer to support other men with prostate cancer through the credo 'Sharing is Caring.' Men get together and talk openly about their fears, and they find that the talk does wonders. Attend an Us Too meeting, and you see men who have shaken off their dread and who are sharing a common bond. The most frequent comment you hear from a first-timer is 'I'm so glad to know I'm not the only one.' Us Too might not be a picture-book retirement package, but I haven't a doubt in my mind that I've enjoyed myself much more than I would have watching the grass grow."

> *Seeing men talk and show compassion for each other has been the antidote to the frustration I felt as a doctor who was taught to envision a man as a collection of organs and glands. It allows me to see a man as a whole.*

US TOO is just one example of men sharing with and caring for each other. Using Us Too as a model, groups meet regularly at the Male Health Center to share their feelings about potency problems, Peyronie's disease (penile curvature), and other male problems.

These support groups demonstrate what I have experienced from helping men with male problems: Men *will* talk sincerely and with feeling if only someone asks them to. In fact, when there are support group meetings, when the Male Health Center holds prostate cancer screenings, or when television crews come to do stories about male health problems, we're overwhelmed with volunteers who want to talk with and help their fellow men. They leave their phone number at the Male Health Center for any man to call and talk. They come to the hospital to visit men who are about to have surgery. They care.

Seeing men talk and show compassion for each other has been the antidote to the frustration I felt as a doctor who was taught to envision a man as a collection of organs and glands. It allows me to see a man as a whole. In the past, I sometimes saw my job as damage control, putting the same men back together over and over again. Today, I see men healing. As a doctor, I help them heal, but they also help each other heal—physically and emotionally.

On occasion, I still have to tell a man that he has prostate cancer and that it has spread, and the hours I spend are sometimes exhausting. But the changes I've seen make it all worth it. Not only are men living longer and better, they're being better partners, fathers and friends.

We have only just started down this road to a new sort of man. There's a long way to go, but there's also a proud and honest precedent set by the hundreds of great men I have had the honor to meet.

Join us. You can make a difference—to you, your partner, your children, and your fellow man.

In health,

Len Goldberg, M.D.

HOTLINES	
Men's Health Network	• (202) 543-6461
National Men's Resource Center	• (415) 453-2839
Us Too Hotline	• (800) 828-7866

A

Prescription Drugs That Might Cause Desire, Potency, or Ejaculatory Problems

High blood Pressure and Antiangial Medications

APPENDIX

Some prescription drugs that might cause desire, potency, or ejaculatory problems (brand names with first word of generic name in brackets):

Many high blood pressure and some antianginal medications might affect potency. See your doctor if you have a problem at the same time as taking some

alpha adrenergic blockers
(Cardura, Dibenzyline, Esimil or Ismelin [guanethidine], Hylorel [guanadrel], Hytrin, Minipress, and Mini-zide);

a medication that contains methyldopa
(Aldoclor, Aldomet, and Aldoril);

andrenergic stimulants
(Catapres [clonidine], Combipres [clonidine and chlorthalidone], Tenex [guanfacine] and Wytensin [guanabenz]);

angiotensin converting enzyme (ACE) inhibitors
(Lotensin [benazepril], Capoten [captopril], and Vasotec [enalapril];

beta blockers
(Blocadren [timolol], Cartrol [carteolol], Corgard [nadolol], Inderal [propranolol], Kerlone [betaxolol], Levatol [penbutolol], Lopressor [meto-

prolol], Sectral [acebutolol], Tenormin [atenolol], Toprol [metoprolol], and Visken [pindolol]),

calcium channel blockers
(Adalat or Procardia [nifedipine], Calan or Isoptin or Verelan [verapamil], Cardene [nicardipine], Cardizem or Dilacor [diltiazem], Dynacirc [isradipine], Norvasc [amlodipine], Plendil [felodipine], and Vascor [bepridil]);

diuretics
(Aldactone [spironoloactone], Bumex [bumetanide], Lozol [indapamide], Midamor [amiloride], and Mykrox or Zaroxolyn [metolazone]);

combination drugs containing reserpine
(Diupres, Hydropres, and Ser-Ap-Es).

Ulcer and Irritable-Bowel-Syndrome Medications	Some ulcer and irritable-bowel-syndrome medications that might affect sexual function include Cantil [mepenzolate], Donnatal, Kinesed [belladonna and phenobarbital], Levsin [hyoscyamine], Pro-Banthine [propantheline], Quarzan [clidinium], Robinul [glycopyrrolate], and Tagamet [cimetidine].
Antianxiety Drugs	Some antianxiety drugs that might cause sexual problems include BuSpar [buspirone], Centrax [prazepam], Limbitrol [chlordiazepoxide and amitriptyline], Valium [diazepam], and Xanax [alprazolam].
Antidepressant Drugs	Most antidepressant drugs can produce sexual difficulties. These might include

amine-oxidase (MAO) inhibitors
(Marplan [isocarboxazid], Nardil [phenelzine], and Parnate [tranylcypromine]);

serotonin-uptake inhibitors
(Prozac [fluoxetine] and Zoloft [ertraline]);

tricyclic antidepressants
(Ludiomil [maprotiline], Adapin [doxepin], Anafranil [clomipramine], Asendin [amoxapine], Elavil and Endep [amitriptyline], Etrafon and Triavil [perphenazine and amitriptyline], Norpramin [desipramine], Pemlor [nortriptyline], Sinequan [doxepin], Surmontil [trimipramine], Tofranil [imipramine], and Vivactil [protriptyline]; Desyrel [trazodone], which might cause ejaculation changes; and Wellbutrin [bupropion]).

Antipsychotics

Most antipsychotics might have some effect on sexual performance, including Clozaril [clozapine], Compazine [prochlorperazine], Haldol [haloperidol], Eskalith, Lithane, Lithium, Lithobid, Lithonate, Lithotabs, or Cibalith-S [lithium], Mellaril [thioridazine], Navane (thiothixene), Prolixin [fluphenazine], Serentil [mesoridazine], Stelazine [trifluoperazine], Taractan [chlorprothixene], Thorazine [chlorpromazine], and Trilafon [perphenazine].

Amphetamine Stimulants

Amphetamine stimulants, such as Desoxyn [methamphetamine], are sometimes prescribed for weight loss and are associated with impotence.

Drug Treatments for Various Diseases and Addictions

Some drug treatments for fhe following ailments may impair the sexual function:

Herion Addiction
Methadone (also called Dolophine), a drug used to help heroin addicts quit, might have effects on erectile ability.

Alcohol Abuse
Antabuse [disulfiram], a drug to help people resist alcohol abuse, might cause impotence in some men.

Tuberculosis
The tubercolosis drug Trecator [ethionamide] has been associated with potency problems in some men.

Insomnia

The insomnia medication Doral [quazepam] has been reported to impede erections in some men.

Prostate Cancer

Any estrogen- or progesterone-containing drug (given to combat prostate cancer) will reduce sexual function.

Glaucoma

The blood pressure medication timolol is also used in eye drops for glaucoma, and might cause erection problems, loss of sex drive, and reduced ejaculate volume when used in this way as well.

B

Resources

APPENDIX

Resources for this book came from a wide variety of sources, including medical journals, personal interviews, and books. Much of that material might be overwhelming to a person without some medical background, but the reader who would like to dig into the subject matter more deeply will find the following titles both readable and informative:

Cooper, Kenneth H., *Controlling Cholesterol*, New York: Bantam Books, 1988.

Connors, Jimmy, *Don't Count Yourself Out*, New York: Hyperion, 1992.

Danoff, Dudley, *Superpotency*, New York: Time-Warner, 1993.

Farrell, Warren, *The Myth of Male Power*, New York: Simon and Schuster, 1993.

Goldstein, Irwin, and Rothstein, Larry, *The Potent Male*, Los Angeles: Price Stern Sloan, Inc., 1990.

Kaplan, Helen Singer, *PE: Overcoming Premature Ejaculation*, New York: Brunner, Mazel, 1989.

LaFavore, Michael, *Men's Health Advisor*, Emmaus, Pennsylvania: Rodale Press, 1992.

Ornish, Dean, *Eat More, Weigh Less*, New York: Harper Collins, 1993.

Zilbergeld, Bernie, *The New Male Sexuality*, Boston: Little, Brown and Company, 1993.